DIABETIC COOKBOOK

for Beginners

1000 Days of Easy, Mouthwatering and Type 2 Diabetes-Friendly Recipes with a Truly Healthy Approach to Life for the Newly Diagnosed.

<u>28-Day Meal Plan Included</u>

LARA RUSH

Table of Contents

INTRODUCTION

What is Diabetes?

Diabetes is a chronic condition affecting how your body regulates blood sugar. There are two main types of diabetes, type 1 and type 2. Type 1 diabetes, also known as juvenile diabetes, is caused by the destruction of insulin-producing cells in the pancreas. Type 2 diabetes is more common and occurs when the body becomes resistant to insulin or doesn't produce enough of it. People with diabetes can have trouble regulating their blood sugar levels, leading to serious health complications such as heart disease, stroke, kidney disease, and nerve damage. Although there is no cure for diabetes, it can be managed through lifestyle changes and medication. With proper treatment, people with diabetes can live long and healthy lives.

What is a Diabetic Diet?

A diabetic diet is a diet that is used by people who have diabetes mellitus or high blood sugar. The body cannot make enough insulin to control the sugar levels. A diabetic diet helps to control the amount of sugar in the blood. A diabetic diet is a dietary plan used by people with diabetes mellitus or high blood glucose to minimize their risk of complications. Complications from diabetes can include heart disease, stroke, kidney failure, nerve damage, and blindness. A diabetic diet is, therefore, essential to help control blood sugar levels and reduce the risk of these complications. The main components of a diabetic diet are healthy eating patterns that include high-fibre carbohydrates, low-fat proteins, and monounsaturated fats. In addition, the diet should be low in calories and sodium and contain plenty of water. Following a diabetic diet can be challenging, but it is important to remember that the goal is to improve your health and quality of life.

Healthy Habits You Can Take to delay the onset of diabetes

There are several different causes of diabetes, but the most common cause is genetics. If you have diabetes in your family history, you are more likely to develop the condition yourself. Other causes of diabetes include obesity, poor diet, insufficient exercise, and certain medical conditions such as PCOS or Cushing's syndrome. In most cases, a combination of factors contributes to the development of diabetes. For example, someone who is overweight and has a family history of diabetes is more likely to develop the condition than someone who is overweight and does not have a family history of diabetes. Diabetes treatment typically includes lifestyle changes such as eating a healthy diet, exercising regularly, and taking medication.

Diabetes is a condition in which your body does not properly process glucose or blood sugar. This can lead to high blood sugar levels, which can damage your organs and cause other health problems. You can take several healthy habits to delay the onset of diabetes or prevent it altogether. These include maintaining a healthy weight, eating a healthy diet, exercising regularly, and avoiding tobacco use. If you have a family history of diabetes, you may also be able to delay the onset of the disease by taking certain medications or getting regular screenings. Taking these steps can help control your blood sugar levels and reduce your risk of developing diabetes.

Requirements of a diabetic diet

A diabetes diet is a healthy-eating plan that's naturally rich in nutrients and low in fat and calories. Key elements are fruits, vegetables and whole grains. A diabetes diet is the best eating plan for almost everyone.

When you have diabetes, your body cannot make or properly use insulin. This leads to high blood sugar levels. A diabetes diet helps keep your blood sugar levels in your target range. This enables you to control your blood sugar levels better. The amount of carbohydrates, fat, and protein you eat depends on many factors, including weight and health goals.

There are different diabetes diets, and each person may respond differently to a specific diabetic diet. A dietitian or doctor can recommend a specific diet for an individual. Individuals with diabetes need to check their blood glucose levels regularly to adjust their diet if necessary. Some foods allowed on a diabetic diet include lean proteins, non-starchy vegetables, whole grains, and healthy fats. Individuals should also limit their intake of sugary foods, processed foods, and Alcohol.

Food list

There are a few superstar foods that are particularly good for people with diabetes, such as:

Beans

Beans are an excellent source of nutrition for diabetics. They are low in sugar and contain complex carbohydrates, which the body slowly breaks down into glucose, helping to regulate blood sugar levels. In addition, beans are a good source of protein, iron, and magnesium. All of these nutrients are essential for maintaining good health, but they are especially important for diabetics.

Green leafy vegetables

While there is no one-size-fits-all diet for diabetics, green leafy vegetables should be included in their meal plan. These nutrient-rich foods can help to regulate blood sugar levels and improve insulin sensitivity. In addition, green leafy vegetables are an excellent source of vitamins, minerals, and antioxidants. They can also help to promote a healthy digestive system and protect against chronic diseases.

Fruits

People with diabetes need to be especially careful about the types of food they eat. While a healthy diet is important for everyone, it's even more crucial for diabetics, as the wrong foods can cause blood sugar levels to spike. That's why it's important to choose fruits that are low in sugar but still high in nutrients. Some great options include berries, melon, and grapefruit. And because they're lower in sugar, they won't cause blood sugar levels to spike like some other fruits can.

Nuts

One type of food that can help diabetics regulate their blood sugar is nuts. Nuts are a good source of protein and healthy fats, which help slow down sugar absorption into the bloodstream. In addition, nuts contain fiber and antioxidants, which can also help to control blood sugar levels. For people with diabetes, incorporating a few handfuls of nuts into their daily diet can be a helpful way to keep blood sugar levels under control.

Whole grains

While many different dietary approaches can help manage diabetes, whole grains have shown promise in controlling blood sugar levels. This is because whole grains are a source of slowly digested carbohydrates, which helps to regulate insulin levels and prevent spikes in blood sugar. Moreover, whole grains are also a good source of fiber, which has been shown to promote satiety and weight loss. This can be a valuable benefit for diabetics, who often need to control their weight to manage their condition. For diabetics, who are at increased risk for certain complications, such as heart disease and stroke, this is an important consideration. Many healthy options are available when choosing whole grains, including quinoa, brown rice, and oats.

Fish

Fish is a low-fat, high-protein food that offers a variety of health benefits. For people with diabetes, fish can be an especially good choice, as it can help to regulate blood sugar levels. Fish is also a good source of omega-3 fatty acids, which have been shown to protect against heart disease. In addition, fish is a good source of vitamin D, essential for bone health. Diabetics should aim to eat fish at least twice a week. When choosing fish, it is important to choose varieties lower in mercury, such as salmon, trout, and herring.

Foods to Avoid

A proper diet is essential for managing diabetes and avoiding potentially serious health complications. Patients should work with a registered dietitian to create a meal plan that satisfies their nutritional needs while limiting foods that can raise blood sugar levels. Patients should avoid processed foods, sugary drinks, and simple carbohydrates. Instead, they should focus on eating lean protein, non-starchy vegetables, and whole grains.

There are certain foods that diabetics should avoid to maintain their health. Sugary drinks, such as soda and juice, are high in carbohydrates and can cause a spike in blood sugar levels. Processed foods, such as white bread and pastries, are also high in carbs and can lead to weight gain, which can be difficult to manage for diabetics. In addition, fried foods and red meat are high in saturated fats and should be avoided. Instead, diabetics should focus on eating plenty of fruits, vegetables, and whole grains. These nutritious foods will help to keep blood sugar levels stable and prevent the complications of diabetes.

7 Tips To Improve And Manage Diabetes Successfully

According to the Centers for Disease Control and Prevention, more than 30 million Americans have diabetes. And while there's no cure for the disease, it can be managed successfully with the help of a healthcare team and some lifestyle changes. Here are seven tips for improving and managing diabetes:

1. Make healthy food choices. Eating a variety of nutritious foods is key to managing diabetes. Choose foods that are low in saturated fat and sugar, and make sure to include plenty of fruits, vegetables, and whole grains.

2. Get regular physical activity. Exercise helps to regulate blood sugar levels and can also help to reduce stress, improve sleep, and boost overall health. Aim for at least 30 minutes of moderate-intensity exercise on most days of the week.

3. Monitor blood sugar levels regularly. Checking blood sugar levels regularly helps to ensure that they remain within a target range. Any changes can then be addressed quickly to avoid potential complications.

4. Take medications as prescribed. Taking diabetes medications exactly as prescribed is important to manage the disease effectively. This includes insulin injections if needed.

5. Reduce stress levels. Stress can cause blood sugar levels to rise, so it's important to find ways to relax and de-stress regularly. Methods such as yoga, meditation, and deep breathing can all help manage stress levels.

6. Quit smoking. Smoking harms overall health and can contribute to complications from diabetes, such as heart disease and stroke. If you smoke, quitting is one of the best things you can do for your health.

7. Get regular medical care. In addition to regularly seeing a healthcare provider for checkups, it's important to see other specialists, such as an endocrinologist or ophthalmologist. Doing so helps ensure that any potential complications are identified and treated quickly.

FAQS

Diabetes is a chronic condition that requires close management. A key component of diabetes management is following a healthy diet. While many different dietary approaches can be helpful for people with diabetes, some common questions come up related to this topic.

First, people often wonder what foods they should eat if they have diabetes. While there is no one-size-fits-all answer to this question, people with diabetes should focus on eating plenty of fruits, vegetables, and whole grains. They should also limit their intake of refined carbohydrates, sugary foods, and saturated fats.

Another common question related to diabetic diet is how much food people should eat. Again, there is no one answer to this question, as it will vary depending on factors such as age, activity level, and medications. However, people with diabetes should generally aim to eat small, frequent meals throughout the day. This can help to maintain blood sugar levels and prevent spikes and dips in blood sugar.

Finally, people often ask if they need to avoid certain foods altogether if they have diabetes. While some foods should be limited (such as those high in sugar or refined carbs), there are no specific foods that need to be avoided completely. Instead, people with diabetes should focus on following a healthy diet that includes a variety of nutrient-rich foods.

Does following a diabetic diet mean complete elimination of sugar?

A strict diabetic diet does not mean eliminating sugar from the diet altogether. You can still enjoy a small-sized serving of your favorite dessert if you have diabetes. The key is moderation. Cut back on the other carbohydrate-containing foods when you want to eat sweets. By doing this, you can still enjoy your favorite treats while controlling your blood sugar levels. Remember to always consult with your doctor or registered dietitian to create a healthy eating plan that is right for you.

Is a diet rich in proteins good for diabetics?

A high protein diet may not be the best option for a diabetic. While protein is essential to a healthy diet, eating too much protein (especially animal protein) can cause insulin resistance, a key factor in diabetes. A healthy balanced diet includes all three macronutrients -protein, carbohydrates and fats- in the right proportions. Too much of any one macronutrient can lead to health problems. For diabetics, it is especially important to monitor protein intake and ensure that they get enough protein without overdoing it. Carbohydrates should also be monitored, as they can cause spikes in blood sugar levels. Fats should also be limited, but some fat is necessary for a healthy diet. By following a balanced diet and monitoring protein intake, diabetics can help to keep their condition under control.

Is it important to maintain a daily intake of carbohydrates?

When you have diabetes, it's important to keep your blood sugar within a target range. That way, you can avoid short- and long-term health problems from highs and lows. A major part of achieving this goal is consistent daily carbohydrate intake. Eating carbohydrates breaks down into sugar (glucose), which raises your blood sugar. If your carb intake is erratic, you may take too much or too little medicine, which can lead to highs or lows. So aim for consistency at every meal and snack, and your blood sugar will thank you.

Can I add ice cream and artificial sweeteners to my diabetic diet?

The short answer is that you can certainly add artificial sweeteners to your diabetic diet, which may even be beneficial in moderation. The main thing to remember is that you should not eat ice cream regularly, as this can offset the benefits of artificial sweeteners. However, moderate use of artificial sweeteners can help diabetics to make their diets more varied and acceptable. Some studies have even shown that sugar-free ice cream can help to improve blood sugar control. Ultimately, speaking with a medical professional before making any significant changes to your diet is important.

<u>What types of foods should they eat if they have diabetes?</u>

While there is no one-size-fits-all answer to this question, people with diabetes should focus on eating plenty of fruits, vegetables, and whole grains. They should also limit their intake of refined carbohydrates, sugary foods, and saturated fats.

BREAKFAST

Recipes

By: Lara Rush

Beet & Strawberry Smoothie Bowl

Servings: 02
Prep time: 10 minutes

Ingredients

- ½ C. beet, peeled and chopped
- ½ C. fresh strawberries
- ½ C. unsweetened almond milk
- 4-6 ice cubes

Directions

1. In a high-power blender, place all ingredients and pulse until creamy.
2. Pour into serving bowls and serve immediately.

Per Serving:

Calories: 40| Fat: 1.1g| Carbs: 7.5g| Fiber: 1.8g| Protein: 1.2g

Berries Yogurt Bowl

Servings: 04
Prep time: 10 minutes

Ingredients

- ¼ C. fresh strawberries, hulled and sliced
- ¼ C. fresh blueberries
- ¼ C. fresh raspberries
- ¼ C. fresh blackberries
- 1 C. fat-free plain Greek yogurt
- 2 tbsp. walnuts, chopped

Directions

1. In a large-sized bowl, blend together the berries.
2. Divide yogurt into serving bowls and top with berries and walnuts.
3. Serve immediately.

Per Serving:

Calories: 172| Fat: 6.6g| Carbs: 15.2g| Fiber: 1.6g | Protein: 10.9g

Blueberry Chia Porridge

Ingredients

- ½ C. frozen blueberries
- 4 tbsp. chia seeds
- 1¼ C. unsweetened almond milk
- ½ tsp. organic vanilla extract
- ½ tbsp. fresh lemon juice
- 3-4 drops liquid stevia

Directions

1. In a high-power blender, add all ingredients and pulse until smooth.

2. Transfer the pudding into two serving bowls and refrigerate to chill before serving.

Per Serving:

Calories: 108| Fat: 7.4g| Carbs: 12.7g| Fiber: 6.5g| Protein: 3.9g

Overnight Oatmeal

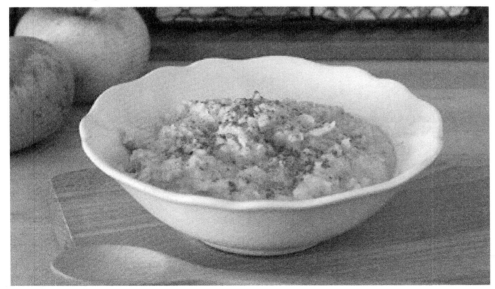

Ingredients

- 1 C. unsweetened almond milk
- 2 tbsp. walnuts, chopped
- 2 tbsp. sunflower seeds

Directions

1. In a saucepan, blend together the milk, walnuts, sunflower seeds, grated apple, vanilla and cinnamon over medium-low heat and cook for about 3-5 minutes.

2. Remove from heat and transfer the porridge into serving

- 1 large apple, peeled, cored and grated
- ½ tsp. organic vanilla extract
- Pinch of ground cinnamon

bowls.

3. Serve warm.

Per Serving:

Calories: 146| Fat: 8g| Carbs: 18g| Fiber: 4.1g| Protein: 3.3g

---

Overnight Oatmeal

Servings: 04

Prep time: 10 minutes

Ingredients

- 2 C. fat-free milk
- 2 C. gluten-free rolled oats
- 1 tsp. lemon zest
- ½ tsp. vanilla extract
- ¼ C. pine nuts
- 2 fresh apricots, chopped
- 2 tbsp. agave nectar

Directions

1. In a large-sized bowl, add milk, oats, lemon zest, and vanilla extract and stir to combine.
2. Cover the bowl and refrigerate overnight.
3. Just before serving, stir in pine nuts, apricots, and agave nectar.

Per Serving:

Calories: 299| Fat: 10.1g| Carbs: 44.3g| Fiber: 5.g| Protein: 10.5g

---

Baked Oatmeal

Servings: 08

Prep time: 15 mins

Cooking Time: 55 mins

Ingredients

- Olive oil cooking spray
- 2 C. gluten-free old-fashioned oats
- ½ C. walnuts, chopped
- 1 tsp. baking powder
- 2 tsp. ground cinnamon
- ¼ tsp. ground nutmeg

Directions

1. Preheat your oven to 375 °F. Grease a 9-inch-square baking dish with cooking spray.
2. In a large-sized bowl, blend together the oats, walnuts, baking powder, spices and salt.
3. In another medium bowl, add almond milk, yogurt, maple syrup, oil, and vanilla extract and beat until well combined.

- ¾ tsp. salt
- 2 C. unsweetened almond milk
- 1 C. fat-free plain Greek yogurt
- ¼ C. maple syrup
- 2 tbsp. extra-virgin olive oil
- 1 tsp. organic vanilla extract
- 2 pears, cored and chopped finely

4. Add the milk mixture into the bowl of oat mixture and mix until well combined.
5. Gently fold in the pear pieces.
6. Place the mixture into the prepared baking dish and spread in an even layer.
7. Bake for approximately 45-55 minutes or until golden brown.
8. Remove the baking dish f oatmeal from oven and set aside to cool before serving.
9. Serve with a splash of your favorite milk.

Per Serving:

Calories: 237| Fat: 10.5g| Carbs: 32.3g| Fiber: 4.7g| Protein: 6.2g

Oat Waffles

Servings: 08

Prep time: 10 minutes

Cooking Time: 40 mins

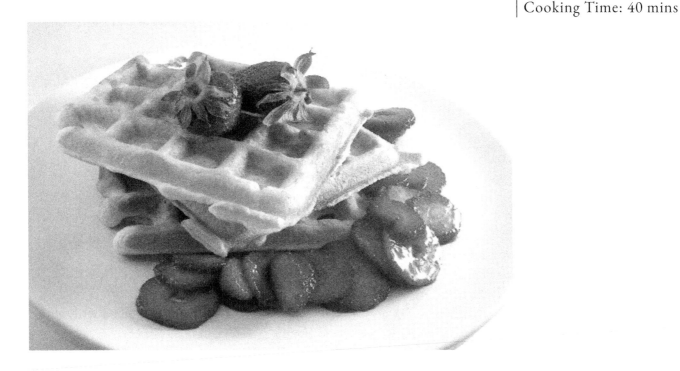

Ingredients

- 1 egg, beaten
- 1¾ C. unsweetened almond milk
- ½ C. unsweetened applesauce

Directions

1. In a large-sized bowl, add egg, almond milk, applesauce, chia seeds, and vanilla extract and beat until well combined.
2. Set aside for about 2 minutes.

- 2 tbsp. chia seeds
- 1 tsp. vanilla extract
- 1¼ C. whole-wheat flour
- ½ C. gluten-free rolled oats
- ¼ C. flaxseed meal
- 4 tsp. baking powder
- 2 tsp. Erythritol
- ¼ tsp. salt
- Olive oil cooking spray

3. In another bowl, blend together the flour, oats, flaxseed meal, baking powder, Erythritol, and salt.
4. Add the flour mixture into the almond milk mixture and beat until smooth.
5. Preheat your waffle iron and then grease it with cooking spray.
6. Place ½ C. of the mixture into preheated waffle iron and cook for about 4-5 minutes or until golden-brown.
7. Repeat with remaining mixture.
8. Serve warm..

Per Serving:

Calories: 176| Fat: 4.1g| Carbs: 29.8g| Fiber: 3.5g| Protein: 5.8g

---

Carrot Muffins

Servings: 06
Prep time: 15 mins
Cooking Time: 17 mins

Ingredients

- Olive oil cooking spray
- 1/3 C. gluten-free rolled oats
- ¼ tsp. baking powder
- 1/8 tsp. baking soda
- ¼ tsp. ground cinnamon
- ¼ tsp. salt
- ¾ C. carrot, peeled and shredded
- 2 small eggs
- 2-3 tbsp. Erythritol
- 3 tbsp. olive oil
- 1 tsp. organic vanilla extract

Directions

1. Preheat your oven to 350 °F. Grease 12 cups of a mini muffin tin.
2. In a blender, add oats and pulse until finely ground.
3. Add baking powder, baking soda, cinnamon and salt and pulse until just combined.
4. Add carrot, eggs, Erythritol, oil and vanilla extract and pulse until smooth.
5. Place the mixture into the prepared muffin cups evenly.
6. Bake for approximately 15-17 minutes or until a wooden skewer inserted in the center comes out clean.
7. Remove the muffin tin from oven and place onto a wire rack to cool for about 10 minutes.
8. Then invert the muffins onto a wire rack to cool completely before serving.

Per Serving:

Calories: 102| Fat: 8.6g| Carbs: 4.7g| Fiber: 0.8g| Protein: 2.2g

Blueberry Pancakes

Servings: 04
Prep time: 10 mins
Cooking Time: 16 mins

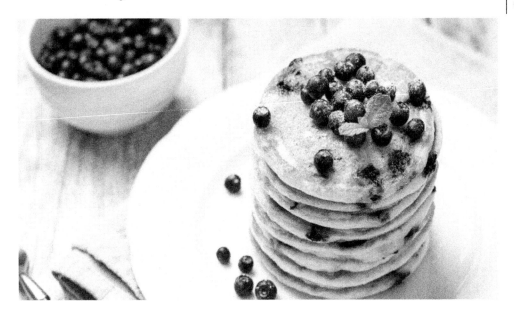

Ingredients

- ½ C. low-fat cottage cheese
- ½ C. gluten-free instant oatmeal
- 2 tbsp. powdered peanuts
- 4 large egg whites
- ½ C. frozen blueberries
- Olive oil cooking spray

Directions

1. In a small-sized blender, add the cottage cheese, oatmeal, powdered peanuts and egg whites and pulse until smooth. (The mixture should be like a pancake batter).
2. Transfer the mixture into a mixing bowl.
3. Gently fold in the blueberries.
4. Lightly grease a non-stick wok with cooking spray and heat over medium heat.
5. Add ¼ of the mixture and with a spoon, spread in an even layer.
6. Cook for about 2 minutes per side or until bottom becomes golden brown.
7. Repeat with remaining mixture.
8. Serve warm.

Per Serving:
Calories: 111| Fat: 3.6g| Carbs: 11.6g| Fiber: 1.9g| Protein: 10.2g

Simple Bread

Servings: 08

Prep time: 10 mins

Cooking Time: 1 hrs 10 mins

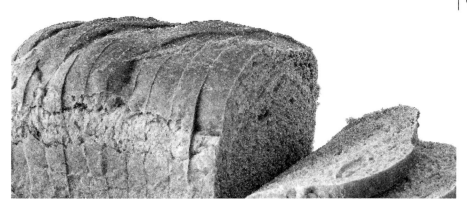

Ingredients

- Olive oil cooking spray
- 4 C. spelt flour
- 4 tbsp. sesame seeds
- 1 tsp. baking soda
- ¼ tsp. salt
- 10-12 drops liquid stevia
- 2 C. plus 2 tbsp. unsweetened almond milk

Directions

1. Preheat your oven to 350 °F. Line a 9x5-inch loaf pan with parchment paper and then grease it with cooking spray.
2. In a large-sized bowl, add all the ingredients and mix until well combined.
3. Transfer the mixture into the prepared loaf pan evenly.
4. Bake for approximately 70 minutes or until a toothpick inserted in the center comes out clean.
5. Remove from oven and place the loaf pan onto a wire rack to cool for at least 10 minutes.
6. Then invert the bread onto the wire rack to cool completely.
7. Cut the bread loaf into desired-sized slices and serve.

Per Serving:
Calories: 239| Fat: 4.2g| Carbs: 45.1g| Fiber: 8.1g| Protein: 9.3g

Spinach Muffins

Servings: 10

Prep time: 10 minutes

Cooking Time: 25 mins

Ingredients

- Olive oil cooking spray
- 1 (10-oz.) package frozen

Directions

1. Preheat your oven to 350 °F. Grease 10 cups of a muffin tin with cooking spray.

- chopped spinach, thawed and drained
- 2 (4-oz.) cartons liquid egg whites
- 6 oz. low-fat sharp cheddar cheese, shredded
- 1 tsp. hot sauce
- 1 tsp. salt
- ½ tsp. ground black pepper

2. In a bowl, add all ingredients and mix until well combined.
3. Place the mixture into the prepared muffin cups evenly.
4. Bake for approximately 20-25 minutes or until top becomes golden brown.
5. Remove the muffin tin from oven and place onto a wire rack to cool for about 10 minutes.
6. Then invert the muffins onto the wire rack and serve warm.

Per Serving:

Calories: 88| Fat: 5.8g| Carbs: 1.3g| Fiber: 0.7g| Protein: 7.5g

Nuts & Seeds Cereal

Servings: 04
Prep time: 10 mins

Ingredients

- ¼ C. almonds, chopped
- ¼ C. walnuts, chopped
- ¼ C. pecans, chopped
- 2 tbsp. mixed seeds
- 2 tbsp. unsweetened coconut flakes, toasted
- 6 fresh strawberries, hulled and sliced
- ¼ C. fresh blueberries
- ½-¾ C. fat-free milk
- 1 tsp. Erythritol

Directions

1. In a large-sized bowl, add nuts, seeds, coconut and berries and mix well.
2. Divide the nut mixture into serving bowls and pour in milk.
3. Sprinkle with Erythritol and serve.

Per Serving:

Calories: 341| Fat: 28.5g| Carbs: 15.4g| Fiber: 5.7g| Protein: 9.4g

French Toast

Servings: 06

Prep time: 15 mins

Cooking Time: 36 mins

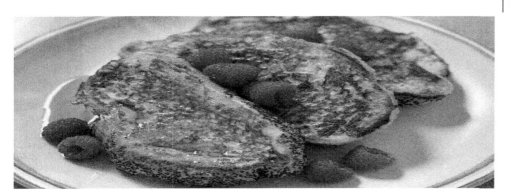

Ingredients

- 1 C. unsweetened almond milk
- 2 tsp. maple syrup
- 1 tsp. organic vanilla extract
- ¼ C. arrowroot starch
- 1 tsp. ground flaxseeds
- ½ tsp. baking powder
- 1 tsp. ground cinnamon
- 2-3 tbsp. coconut oil
- 6 whole-wheat bread slices

Directions

1. In a shallow bowl, whisk together the almond milk, maple syrup, vanilla extract, arrowroot starch, ground flaxseeds, baking powder and cinnamon until well blended.
2. In a non-stick wok, melt a little coconut oil over medium-high heat.
3. Dip both sides of 1 bread slice in milk mixture and cook in the wok for about 3 minutes per side.
4. Repeat with remaining slices.
5. Serve warm.

Per Serving:

Calories: 132| Fat: 6.4g| Carbs: 17.7g| Fiber: 2.3g| Protein: 3.5g

---

Avocado Toast

Servings: 02

Prep time: 10 mins

Cooking Time: 5 mins

Ingredients

- 2 whole-grain bread slices
- ½ avocado, peeled and pitted
- 2 tbsp. fresh cilantro, chopped

Directions

1. Heat a non-stick frying pan over medium heat and toast the bread slices for about 3-5 minutes or until desired doneness, flipping once halfway through.
2. Remove the bread slices from heat and place onto serving plates.
3. Meanwhile, in a bowl, add avocado flesh and with a fork

- 1 tsp. fresh lemon juice
- ¼ tsp. lemon zest, grated
- Pinch of cayenne powder
- Pinch of salt

mash well.

4. Add in cilantro, lemon juice, zest, cayenne powder and salt and stir to combine.

5. Spread avocado mixture onto each bread slice and serve.

Per Serving:

Calories: 175| Fat: 11.2g| Carbs: 16.1g| Fiber: 5.3g| Protein: 3.7g

Poached Eggs With Toast

Servings: 04
Prep time: 10 mins
Cooking Time: 5 mins

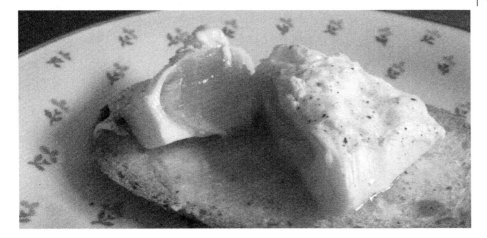

Ingredients

- 4 eggs
- 2 tsp. white vinegar
- Salt and ground black pepper, as required
- Pinch of dried dill
- 4 whole-grain bread slices, toasted

Directions

1. In a large-sized saucepan, add about 2-3-inch of water over medium heat and bring to a simmer.
2. Adjust the heat to medium-low and pour in vinegar.
3. Crack an egg into a small-sized cup.
4. Gently drop the egg into the water.
5. Repeat with remaining eggs.
6. Immediately cover the pan and turn off the heat.
7. Let it sit for about 4 minutes.
8. With a slotted spoon, transfer the eggs onto serving plates.
9. Sprinkle with salt, black pepper, and dill and serve alongside the bread slices.

Per Serving:

Calories: 135| Fat: 5.7g| Carbs: 12g| Fiber: 1.8g| Protein: 8.2g

Oats & Quinoa Granola

Ingredients

- 1 C. gluten-free quick-cooking steel-cut oats
- ½ C. uncooked quinoa, rinsed
- ½ C. walnuts, chopped roughly
- ¼ C. chia seeds
- 1/8 tsp. salt
- 3 tbsp. maple syrup
- 3 tbsp. avocado oil
- 1 tsp. organic vanilla extract
- ¼ C. unsweetened coconut flakes

Directions

1. Preheat your oven to 325 °F. Arrange a rack on a third rack from the bottom of oven.
2. Line a baking sheet with parchment paper.
3. In a medium-sized bowl, add oats, quinoa, walnuts, chia seeds and salt.
4. Add maple syrup, oil and vanilla extract and mix well.
5. Transfer the oat mixture onto the prepared baking sheet and spread in an even layer.
6. Bake for approximately 25 minutes.
7. Sprinkle the top of the granola with coconut flakes and bake for approximately 5 minutes more.
8. Remove from oven and set aside to cool completely.
9. Break the granola into pieces and serve with your favorite milk and topping.

Per Serving:

Calories: 115| Fat: 6.4g| Carbs: 12.5g| Fiber: 2.5g| Protein: 3.5g

---

Kale & Cheddar Omelet

Ingredients

- 4 large eggs
- ½ C. cooked kale, squeezed
- 4 scallions, chopped
- 2 tbsp. fresh parsley, chopped
- ¼ C. low-fat cheddar cheese, shredded
- Salt and ground black pepper, as required
- 2 tsp. olive oil

Directions

1. Preheat the broiler of oven. Arrange a rack about 4-inch from heating element.
2. In a bowl, crack the eggs and beat well.
3. Add remaining ingredients except oil and stir to combine.
4. In an oven-proof wok, heat oil over medium heat.
5. Add egg mixture and tilt the wok to spread the mixture evenly.
6. Immediately, Adjust the heat to medium-low and cook for about 3-4 minutes or until golden brown.
7. Now, transfer the wok under broiler and broil for about

1½-2½ minutes.

8. Serve hot.

Per Serving:

Calories: 247| Fat: 17.5g| Carbs: 5.5g| Fiber: 1.2g| Protein: 17.7g

---

Mushrooms & Eggs Scramble

Servings: 02

Prep time: 10 mins

Cooking Time: 10 mins

Ingredients

- 2 large eggs
- 2 large egg whites
- Salt and ground black pepper, as required
- 2 tsp. olive oil
- 1 C. fresh mushrooms, sliced thinly
- 2 tbsp. low-fat cheddar cheese, shredded

Directions

1. In a small-sized bowl, add the eggs, egg whites, salt and black pepper and beat until well combined.
2. In a small-sized non-stick wok, heat the oil over medium-high heat cook the mushrooms for about 6-7 minutes.
3. Reduce heat to medium.
4. Add the egg mixture and cook for about 3 minutes, stirring continuously.
5. Stir in the cheese and remove from heat
6. Serve immediately.

Per Serving:

Calories: 159| Fat: 11.3g| Carbs: 2g| Fiber: 0.4g| Protein: 13g

---

Eggs With Tomatoes

Servings: 04

Prep time: 10 mins

Cooking Time: 33 mins

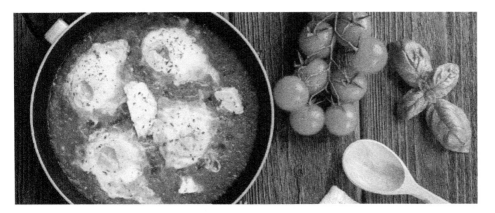

Ingredients

Directions

- 2 tbsp. olive oil
- 4 small yellow onions, sliced thinly
- ½-¾ C. tomatoes, chopped finely
- 1 garlic clove, minced
- 4 large eggs
- 3 oz. low-fat feta cheese, crumbled
- Salt and ground black pepper, as required
- 2 tbsp. fresh parsley, minced

1. In a large-sized cast-iron wok, heat oil over medium-low heat and cook the onions for about 10-15 minutes, stirring occasionally.
2. Add the tomatoes and garlic and cook for about 2-3 minutes, stirring frequently.
3. Adjust the heat to low and with the spoon, spread the mixture in an even layer.
4. Carefully crack the eggs over onion mixture and sprinkle with the feta cheese, salt, and black pepper.
5. Cover the wok tightly and cook for about 10-15 minutes or until desired doneness of the eggs.
6. Serve hot with the garnishing of the parsley.

Per Serving:

Calories: 203| Fat: 14.4g| Carbs: 8.9g| Fiber: 1.9g| Protein: 11.2g

---

Veggie Frittata

Servings: 04
Prep time: 15 mins
Cooking Time: 7 mins

Ingredients

- 1 tbsp. olive oil
- 1 C. frozen mixed veggies (broccoli, cauliflower, and carrot), roughly chopped
- 2 scallions (green and white parts separated), thinly sliced
- Salt, as required
- 2 large eggs, lightly beaten
- 2 tbsp. low-fat cheddar cheese, shredded

Directions

1. In a small-sized non-stick wok, heat oil over medium-high heat and cook the frozen veggies and scallion whites for about 3-5 minutes, stirring occasionally.
2. Stir in scallion greens and pour in eggs.
3. Cook for about 1-2 minutes.
4. Sprinkle with cheese and immediately cover the wok tightly.
5. Remove from heat and set aside, covered for about 4-5 minutes.
6. Divide the frittata in 2 portions and serve.

Per Serving:

Calories: 218| Fat: 13.6g| Carbs: 13.7g| Fiber: 4.4g| Protein: 11.2g

LUNCH

Recipes

By: Lara Rush

Cucumber & Tomato Salad

Servings: 04
Prep time: 15 mins

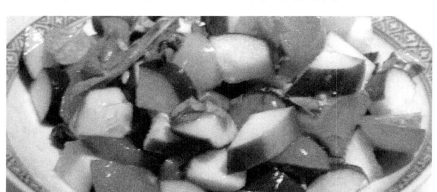

Ingredients

- 2 C. tomatoes, chopped
- 2 C. cucumbers, chopped
- 4 C. fresh baby spinach
- 2 tbsp. olive oil
- 2 tbsp. fresh lemon juice
- Salt, as required

Directions

1. Place all the ingredients in a large-sized serving bowl and gently toss to combine.
2. Serve immediately.

Per Serving:

Calories: 96| Fat: 7.4g| Carbs: 7.9g| Fiber: 1.8g| Protein: 2g

---

Berries & Arugula Salad

Servings: 04
Prep time: 15 minutes

Ingredients

- 1 C. fresh strawberries, hulled and sliced
- ½ C. fresh blackberries
- ½ C. fresh blueberries
- ½ C. fresh raspberries
- 6 C. fresh arugula
- 2 tbsp. extra-virgin olive oil
- Salt and ground black pepper, as required

Directions

1. In a salad bowl, place all the ingredients and toss to coat well.
2. Serve immediately..

Per Serving:

Calories: 105| Fat: 7.6g| Carbs: 10.1g| Fiber: 3.6g| Protein: 1.6g

Green Beans Salad

Ingredients

For Dressing

- 2 tsp. whole-grain mustard
- 2 tbsp. fresh lemon juice
- 2 tbsp. extra-virgin olive oil
- 1 small garlic clove, finely grated
- Salt and ground black pepper, as required

For Salad

- 1 tbsp. olive oil
- 10 oz. fresh green beans, trimmed and sliced
- 1 garlic clove, sliced thinly
- 2 ripe tomatoes, chopped
- 1 C. cherry tomatoes, sliced
- 1 large cucumber, sliced
- 1 small red onion, finely chopped
- 2 C. lettuce, torn
- 2 C. fresh arugula

Directions

1. For dressing: in a bowl, add all ingredients and whisk until well blended. Set aside.
2. In a wok, heat oil over medium-high heat and cook the green beans and garlic for about 5 minutes, stirring frequently.
3. Transfer the green beans into a salad bowl and set aside to cool.
4. Add remaining ingredients and mix well.
5. Drizzle with dressing and serve.

Per Serving:

Calories: 161| Fat: 11.2g| Carbs: 15.4g| Fiber: 4.9g| Protein: 3.6g

Apple & Pear Salad

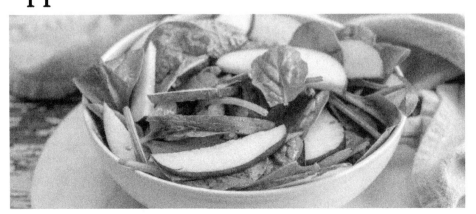

Ingredients

- 2 large apples, cored and sliced
- 2 large pears, cored and sliced
- 6 C. fresh baby spinach
- 3 tbsp. extra-virgin olive oil
- 2 tbsp. apple cider vinegar

Directions

1. In a large-sized bowl, add all the ingredients and toss to coat well.
2. Serve immediately.

Per Serving:

Calories: 218| Fat: 11.1g| Carbs: 32.5g| Fiber: 6.4g| Protein: 1.9g

Chicken Lettuce Wraps

Servings: 05
Prep time: 15 mins
Cooking Time: 15 mins

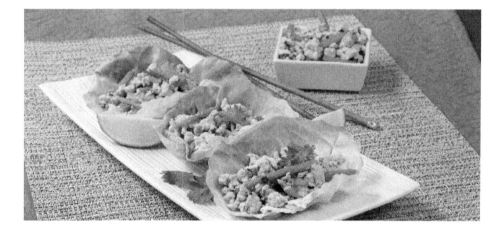

Ingredients

For Chicken

- 2 tbsp. avocado oil
- 1 small onion, chopped finely
- 1 tsp. fresh ginger, minced
- 2 garlic cloves, minced
- 1¼ lb. ground chicken
- Salt and ground black pepper, as required

For Wraps

- 10 romaine lettuce leaves
- 1½ C. carrot, peeled and julienned
- 2 tbsp. fresh parsley, chopped finely

Directions

1. In a wok, heat the oil over medium heat and sauté the onion, ginger, and garlic for about 4-5 minutes.
2. Add the ground chicken, salt, and black pepper, and cook over medium-high heat for about 7-9 minutes, breaking up the meat into smaller pieces with a wooden spoon.
3. Remove from heat and set aside to cool.
4. Arrange the lettuce leaves onto serving plates.
5. Place the cooked chicken over each lettuce leaf and top with carrot and cilantro.
6. Drizzle with lime juice and serve immediately.

• 2 tbsp. fresh lime juice

Per Serving:

Calories: 246| Fat: 9.2g| Carbs: 5.8g| Fiber: 1.5g| Protein: 33.5g

---

Shrimp Lettuce Wraps

Servings: 04
Prep time: 15 mins
Cooking Time: 5 mins

Ingredients

- 1 tsp. olive oil
- 1 garlic clove, minced
- 1½ lb. shrimp, peeled, deveined and chopped
- Salt, as required
- 8 large lettuce leaves
- 1 C. carrot, peeled and julienned
- 1 C. cucumber, julienned
- 1 tbsp. fresh chives, minced

Directions

1. In a large-sized sauté pan, heat the olive oil over medium heat and sauté garlic for about 1 minute.
2. Add the shrimp and cook for about 3-4 minutes.
3. Remove from heat and set aside to cool slightly.
4. Arrange lettuce leaves onto serving plates.
5. Divide the shrimp, carrot and cucumber over the leaves evenly.
6. Garnish with chives and serve immediately.

Per Serving:

Calories: 230| Fat: 4.1g| Carbs: 6.8g| Fiber: 0.9g| Protein: 39.3g

---

Chicken Burgers

Servings: 04
Prep time: 10 mins
Cooking Time: 10 mins

Ingredients

- Olive oil cooking spray
- 1 (½-inch) piece fresh ginger, grated
- ½ lb. lean ground turkey
- ½ of medium onion, grated
- 1 garlic clove, minced
- 1 tsp. fresh mint leaves,

Directions

1. Preheat the broiler of oven. Lightly grease a broiler pan with cooking spray.
2. In a bowl, squeeze the juice of ginger .
3. Add the remaining ingredients except for spinach and mix until well combined.
4. Shape the mixture into 2 equal-sized patties.
5. Arrange the patties onto the prepared broiler pan and

chopped finely
- ½ tsp. ground cumin
- ¼ tsp. paprika
- Salt and ground black pepper, as required
- 2 C. fresh baby spinach

broil for about 5 minutes per side.

6. Serve hot alongside the spinach.

Per Serving:

Calories: 185| Fat: 8.4g| Carbs: 4.6g| Fiber: 1.5g| Protein: 23.7g

Beef Burgers

Servings: 04
Prep time: 15 mins
Cooking Time: 14 mins

Ingredients

- 1½ lb. lean ground beef
- Salt and ground black pepper, as required
- 2 C. fresh spinach
- ½ C. part-skim mozzarella cheese, shredded
- 2 tbsp. low-fat Parmesan cheese, grated
- 4 C. fresh baby arugula

Directions

1. In a bowl, add the beef, salt and black pepper and mix until well combined.
2. Make 8 equal-sized patties from the mixture.
3. Arrange the patties onto a plate and refrigerate until using.
4. In a frying pan, add the spinach over medium-high heat and cook, covered for about 2 minutes or until wilted.
5. Drain the spinach and set aside to cool.
6. With your hands, squeeze the spinach to extract the liquid completely.
7. Place the spinach to a cutting board and then chop it.
8. In a bowl, add the chopped spinach and both cheese and mix well.
9. Place about ¼ C. of the spinach mixture in the center of 4 patties and top each with the remaining 4 patties.
10. With your fingers, press the edges firmly to seal the filling.
11. Then, press each patty slightly to flatten.
12. Heat a lightly greased grill pan over medium-high heat and cook the patties for about 5-6 minutes per side.
13. Serve hot alongside the arugula.

Per Serving:

Calories: 268| Fat: 13.5g| Carbs: 1.4g| Fiber: 0.7g | Protein: 35.9g

---

Pumpkin Soup

Servings: 02
Prep time: 15 minutes
Cooking Time: 25 mins

Ingredients

- 2 tsp. olive oil
- 1 onion, chopped
- 1 tsp. fresh ginger, chopped
- 2 garlic cloves, chopped
- 2 tbsp. fresh cilantro, chopped
- 3 C. pumpkin, peeled and cubed
- 4¼ C. homemade vegetable broth
- Salt and ground black pepper, as required
- ½ C. coconut cream
- 2 tbsp. fresh lime juice

Directions

1. In a large-sized soup pan, heat oil over medium heat and sauté the onion, turmeric, ginger, garlic and cilantro for about 3-4 minutes.
2. Add the pumpkin and broth and bring to a boil
3. Turn the heat to low and simmer, covered for about 15 minutes.
4. Remove from heat and set aside to cool slightly.
5. Transfer the mixture into a high-power blender in batches with avocado and pulse until smooth.
6. Return the soup into the pan over medium heat and cook for 3 minutes or until hot enough.
7. Serve hot.

Per Serving:
Calories: 208| Fat: 11.5g| Carbs: 21g| Fiber: 6.7g| Protein: 8.3g

---

Beans & Walnut Burgers

Servings: 08
Prep time: 20 mins
Cooking Time: 25 mins

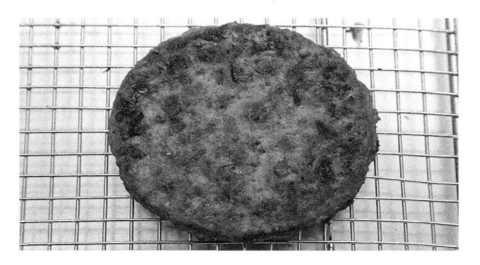

Ingredients

- ½ C. walnuts
- 1 carrot, peeled and chopped
- 1 celery stalk, chopped
- 4 scallions, chopped
- 5 garlic cloves, chopped
- 2¼ C. cooked black beans
- 2½ C. sweet potato, peeled and grated
- ½ tsp. red pepper flakes, crushed
- ¼ tsp. cayenne powder
- Salt and ground black pepper, as required
- 8 C. lettuce, torn

Directions

1. Preheat your oven to 400 °F. Line a baking sheet with parchment paper.
2. In a food processor, add the walnuts and pulse until finely ground.
3. Add the carrot, celery, scallion and garlic and pulse until chopped finely.
4. Transfer the vegetable mixture into a large-sized bowl.
5. In the same food processor, add the beans and pulse until chopped.
6. Add 1½ C. of the sweet potato and pulse until a chunky mixture forms.
7. Transfer the bean mixture into the bowl with vegetable mixture.
8. Stir in remaining sweet potato and spices and mix until well combined.
9. Make 8 equal-sized patties from the mixture.
10. Arrange the patties onto the prepared baking sheet in a single layer.
11. Bake for approximately 25 minutes.
12. Serve hot alongside the lettuce.

Per Serving:

Calories: 300| Fat: 5.5g| Carbs: 49.8g| Fiber: 11.4g| Protein: 15.3g

Pumpkin Soup

Servings: 04
Prep time: 15 mins
Cooking Time: 25 mins

Ingredients

- 2 tsp. olive oil
- 1 onion, chopped
- 1 tsp. fresh ginger, chopped
- 2 garlic cloves, chopped
- 2 tbsp. fresh cilantro, chopped
- 3 C. pumpkin, peeled and cubed
- 4¼ C. homemade vegetable

Directions

1. In a large-sized soup pan, heat oil over medium heat and sauté the onion, turmeric, ginger, garlic and cilantro for about 3-4 minutes.
2. Add the pumpkin and broth and bring to a boil
3. Turn the heat to low and simmer, covered for about 15 minutes.
4. Remove from heat and set aside to cool slightly.
5. Transfer the mixture into a high-power blender in batches

broth
- Salt and ground black pepper, as required
- ½ C. coconut cream
- 2 tbsp. fresh lime juice

with avocado and pulse until smooth.

6. Return the soup into the pan over medium heat and cook for 3 minutes or until hot enough.

7. Serve hot.

Per Serving:

Calories: 208| Fat: 11.5g| Carbs: 21g| Fiber: 6.7g| Protein: 8.3g

Mushrooms With Bok Choy

Servings: 04
Prep time: 15 mins
Cooking Time: 10 mins

Ingredients

- 1 lb. baby bok choy
- 4 tsp. olive oil
- 1 tsp. fresh ginger, minced
- 2 garlic cloves, chopped
- 5 oz. fresh mushrooms, sliced
- 2 tbsp. homemade chicken broth
- 2 tbsp. low-sodium soy sauce
- Ground black pepper, as required

Directions

1. Trim bases of bok choy and separate outer leaves from stalks, leaving the smallest inner leaves attached.

2. In a large-sized cast-iron wok, heat the oil over medium-high heat and sauté the ginger and garlic for about 1 minute.

3. Stir in the mushrooms and cook for about 4-5 minutes, stirring frequently.

4. Stir in the bok choy leaves and stalks and cook for about 1 minute, tossing with tongs.

5. Stir in the broth, soy sauce and black pepper and cook for about 2-3 minutes, tossing occasionally.

6. Serve hot.

Per Serving:

Calories: 77| Fat: 5g| Carbs: 5.3g| Fiber: 1.6g| Protein: 3.5g

Broccoli Soup

Servings: 04

Prep time: 15 mins

Cooking Time: 45 mins

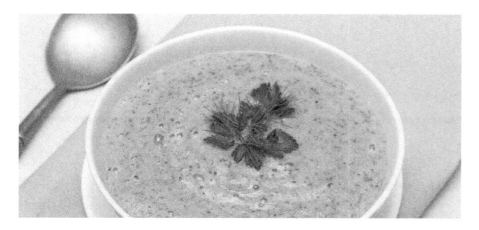

Ingredients

- 2 tbsp. olive oil
- ½ C. onion, chopped
- 1 garlic clove, minced
- 1 tbsp. fresh thyme, chopped
- ¼ tsp. ground cumin
- ¼ tsp. red pepper flakes, crushed
- 2 medium heads broccoli, cut into florets
- 4 C. homemade vegetable broth
- 1 avocado, peeled, pitted and chopped

Directions

1. In a large-sized soup pan, heat the oil over medium heat and sauté the onion for about 4-5 minutes.
2. Add the garlic, thyme and spices and sauté for about 1 minute more.
3. Add the broccoli and cook for about 3-4 minutes.
4. Stir in the broth and bring to a boil over high heat.
5. Adjust the heat to medium-low.
6. Cover the soup pan and cook for 32-35 minutes.
7. Remove from heat and set aside to cool slightly.
8. In a blender, place the mixture in batches with avocado and pulse until smooth.
9. Serve immediately.

Per Serving:

Calories: 254| Fat: 18.7g| Carbs: 15.8g| Fiber: 7.3g| Protein: 9.7g

Tofu With Kale

Servings: 02
Prep time: 15 mins
Cooking Time: 10 mins

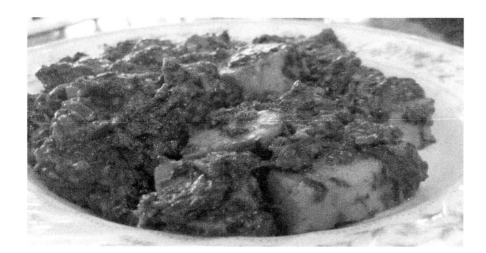

Ingredients

- 1 tbsp. olive oil
- ½ lb. tofu, pressed, drained and cubed
- 1 tsp. fresh ginger, minced
- 1 garlic clove, minced
- ¼ tsp. red pepper flakes, crushed
- 6 oz. fresh kale, tough ribs removed and chopped finely
- 1 tbsp. low-sodium soy sauce

Directions

1. Heat the olive oil in a large-sized non-stick wok over medium-high heat and stir-fry the tofu for about 3-3 minutes.
2. Add the ginger, garlic and red pepper flakes and cook for about 1 minute, stirring continuously.
3. Stir in the kale and soy sauce and stir-fry for about 4-5 minutes.
4. Serve hot.

Per Serving:
Calories: 190| Fat: 11.8g| Carbs: 12.6g| Fiber: 2.5g| Protein: 12.5g

Stuffed Zucchini

Servings: 08
Prep time: 15 mins
Cooking Time: 18 mins

Ingredients

- Olive oil cooking spray
- 4 medium zucchinis, halved lengthwise
- 1 C. red bell pepper,

Directions

1. Preheat your oven to 350 °F. Grease a large-sized baking sheet with cooking spray.
2. With a melon baller, scoop out the flesh of each zucchini half. Discard the flesh.

- seeded and minced
- ½ C. Kalamata olives, pitted and minced
- ½ C. fresh tomatoes, minced
- 1 tsp. garlic, minced
- 1 tbsp. dried oregano, crushed
- Salt and ground black pepper, as required
- ½ C. low-fat feta cheese, crumbled

3. In a bowl, blend together the bell pepper, olives, tomatoes, garlic, oregano, salt and black pepper.
4. Stuff each zucchini half evenly with the veggie mixture.
5. Arrange zucchini halves onto the prepared baking sheet and bake for approximately 15 minutes.
6. Now, set the oven to broiler on high.
7. Top each zucchini half with feta cheese and broil for about 3 minutes.
8. Serve hot.

Per Serving:
Calories: 59| Fat: 3.2g| Carbs: 6.2g| Fiber: 0.9g| Protein: 2.9g

Lentil & Rice Loaf

Servings: 04
Prep time: 20 mins
Cooking Time: 1 hrs 50 mins

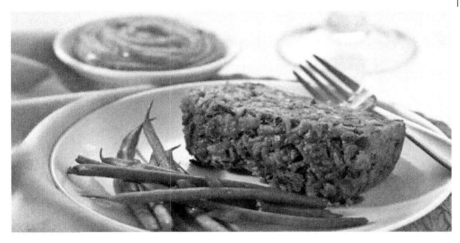

Ingredients

- 1¾ C. plus 2 tbsp. water, divided
- ½ C. wild rice
- ½ C. brown lentils
- Salt, as required
- ½ tsp. Italian seasoning
- 1 medium yellow onion, chopped
- 1 celery stalk, chopped

Directions

1. In a saucepan, add 1¾ C. of the water, rice, lentils, salt and Italian seasoning over medium-high heat and bring to a rolling boil.
2. Adjust the heat to low and cook, covered for about 45 minutes.
3. Remove the pan from heat and set aside, covered for at least 10 minutes.
4. Preheat your oven to 350 °F and line a 9x5-inch loaf pan with parchment paper.

- 6 cremini mushrooms, chopped
- 4 garlic cloves, minced
- ¾ C. gluten-free rolled oats
- ½ C. walnuts, chopped finely
- ¾ C. sugar-free ketchup
- ½ tsp. red pepper flakes, crushed
- 1 tsp. fresh rosemary, minced
- 2 tsp. fresh thyme, minced

5. In a wok, heat the remaining water over medium heat and sauté the onion, celery, mushrooms and garlic for about 4-5 minutes.
6. Remove from heat and set aside to cool slightly.
7. In a large-sized bowl, add the oats, walnuts, ketchup and fresh herbs and mix until well combined.
8. Add the rice mixture and vegetable mixture and mix well.
9. In a blender, add the mixture and pulse until just a chunky mixture forms.
10. Place the mixture into the prepared loaf pan evenly.
11. With a piece of foil, cover the loaf pan and bake for approximately 40 minutes.
12. Uncover and bake for 20 minutes more or until top becomes golden brown.
13. Remove from oven and place the loaf pan onto a wire rack for about 10 minutes.
14. Carefully invert the loaf onto a platter.
15. Cut into desired-sized slices and serve.

Per Serving:
Calories: 254| Fat: 7.5g| Carbs: 38.6g| Fiber: 8.5g| Protein: 11.5g

---

Turkey Meatloaf

Servings: 04
Prep time: 15 mins
Cooking Time: 43 mins

Ingredients

- 2 tsp. olive oil
- ½ C. red onion, chopped
- 1 tsp. garlic, minced
- 1 lb. lean ground turkey
- 1/3 C. low-fat feta cheese, crumbled
- ¼ C. whole-wheat breadcrumbs
- ½ C. roasted red peppers, chopped
- ¼ C. green olives, pitted and chopped
- 1 tbsp. fresh dill, chopped
- 2 tbsp. fresh parsley,

Directions

1. Preheat your oven to 400 °F. Line a baking sheet with parchment paper.
2. In a non-stick wok, heat the oil over medium heat and sauté the onion for about 2 minutes.
3. Add the garlic and sauté for 1 minute.
4. Remove from heat and transfer the mixture into a large-sized mixing bowl.
5. In the bowl, add the remaining ingredients and with your hands, mix until well combined.
6. Place the mixture onto the prepared baking sheet and with your hands, shape into a loaf.
7. Bake for approximately 30-40 minutes.

chopped

- 2 tsp. dried oregano
- Salt and ground black pepper, as required
- 1 egg
- 1 tbsp. fat-free milk

8. Remove from oven and place the meatloaf aside for about 10 minutes before serving.
9. Cut the meatloaf into desired-sized slices and serve..

Per Serving:

Calories: 283| Fat: 14.8g| Carbs: 6.4g| Fiber: 1.4g | Protein: 26.5g

Garlicky Shrimp

Servings: 02
Prep time: 15 mins
Cooking Time: 6 mins

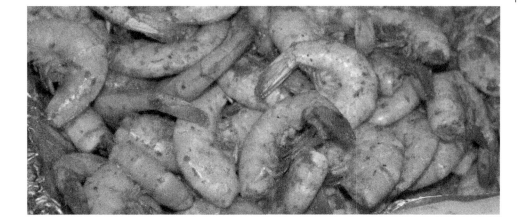

Ingredients

- 1 tbsp. olive oil
- 2 garlic cloves, minced
- 1 tbsp. fresh parsley, chopped
- ½ lb. shrimp, peeled and deveined
- 2 tbsp. water
- Salt and ground black pepper, as required

Directions

1. In a large-sized wok, heat the oil over medium heat and sauté the garlic and parsley for about 1 minute.
2. Stir in the shrimp, water, salt and black pepper and cook for about 4-5 minutes or until done completely.
3. Serve hot.

Per Serving:

Calories: 200| Fat: 9g| Carbs: 2.8g| Fiber: 0.1g| Protein: 26.1g

Shrimp With Kale

Servings: 04
Prep time: 15 mins
Cooking Time: 10 mins

Ingredients

- 3 tbsp. olive oil
- 1 lb. medium shrimp, peeled and deveined
- 1 medium onion, chopped
- 4 garlic cloves, chopped finely
- 1 fresh red chili, sliced
- 1 lb. fresh kale, tough ribs removed and chopped
- ¼ C. homemade chicken broth

Directions

1. In a large-sized non-stick wok, heat 1 tbsp. of the oil over medium-high heat and cook the shrimp for about 2 minutes per side.
2. With a slotted spoon, transfer the shrimp onto a plate.
3. In the same wok, heat the remaining 2 tbsp. of oil over medium heat and sauté the garlic and red chili for about 1 minute.
4. Add the kale and broth and cook for about 4-5 minutes, stirring occasionally.
5. Stir in the cooked shrimp and cook for about 1 minute.
6. Serve hot.

Per Serving:

Calories: 270| Fat: 11.9g| Carbs: 15.5g| Fiber: 2.3g| Protein: 28.3g

---

Scallops With Broccoli

Servings: 02
Prep time: 15 mins
Cooking Time: 9 mins

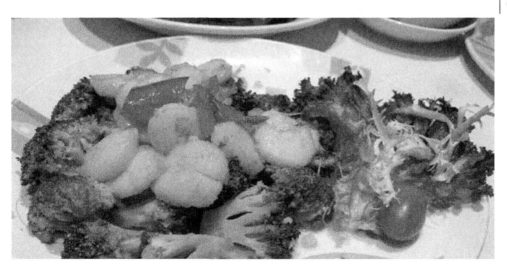

Ingredients

- 2 tbsp. olive oil

Directions

1. Heat oil in a large-sized cast-iron wok over medium heat

- 1 C. broccoli, cut into small pieces
- 1 garlic clove, crushed
- ½ lb. sea scallops, side muscle removed
- 1 tsp. fresh lemon juice
- Salt, as required

and cook the broccoli and garlic for about 3-4 minutes, stirring occasionally.

2. Add in the scallops and cook for about 3-4 minutes, flipping occasionally.
3. Stir in the lemon juice and remove from heat.
4. Serve hot.

Per Serving:

Calories: 220| Fat: 12.6g| Carbs: 6.3g| Fiber: 1.2g| Protein: 20.5g

Scallops With Spinach

Servings: 04
Prep time: 15 mins
Cooking Time: 10 mins

Ingredients

- 20 oz. sea scallops, side muscle removed
- Salt and ground black pepper, as required
- 3 tsp. olive oil, divided
- 6 oz. fresh baby spinach
- 2 garlic cloves, minced
- 1 tbsp. fresh lemon juice

Directions

1. Season the scallops with salt and black pepper evenly.
2. In a large-sized cast-iron wok, heat 2 tsp. of oil over medium heat and cook the scallops for about 2-3 minutes per side.
3. With a slotted spoon, transfer the scallops onto a plate.
4. In the same wok, heat remaining oil over medium heat and cook the spinach and garlic for about 3-4 minutes.
5. Stir in the salt and black pepper and remove from heat.
6. Transfer the spinach onto serving plates and top with scallops.
7. Drizzle with lemon juice and serve.

Per Serving:

Calories: 165| Fat: 4.4g| Carbs: 5.5g| Fiber: 1g| Protein: 25.2g

DINNER

Recipes

By: Lara Rush

Chickpeas & Quinoa Salad

Servings: 06
Prep time: 20 mins
Cooking Time: 20 mins

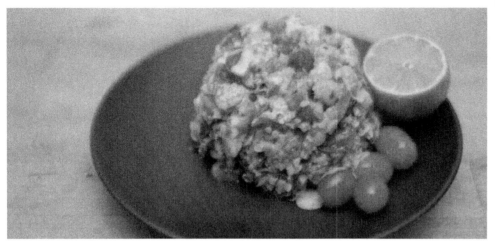

Ingredients

- 1¾ C. homemade vegetable broth
- 1 C. quinoa, rinsed
- Sea salt, as required
- 1½ C. cooked chickpeas
- 2 medium bell peppers, seeded and chopped
- 2 cucumbers, chopped
- ½ C. scallion (green part), chopped
- 1 tbsp. olive oil
- 2 tbsp. fresh parsley leaves, chopped

Directions

1. In a saucepan, add the broth over high heat and bring to a boil.
2. Add the quinoa and salt and cook until boiling.
3. Adjust the heat to low and simmer, covered for about 15-20 minutes or until all the liquid is absorbed.
4. Remove from heat and set aside, covered for about 5-10 minutes.
5. Uncover and with a fork, fluff the quinoa.
6. In a large-sized serving bowl, place the quinoa with the remaining ingredients and gently toss to coat.
7. Serve immediately.

Per Serving:

Calories: 348| Fat: 7.7g| Carbs: 56g| Fiber: 11.9g| Protein: 16.3g

Lentil Salad

Servings: 02
Prep time: 15 mins
Cooking Time: 7 mins

Ingredients

- ½ tbsp. plus 1 tsp. olive oil

Directions

1. In a small-sized bowl, whisk together ½ tbsp. olive oil,

- 3 tbsp. balsamic vinegar
- 1 tbsp. Dijon mustard
- 1 ½ tsp. Herbs de Provence
- Salt and ground black pepper, as required
- 1 clove garlic, minced
- 1 C. cooked lentils
- 1 large carrot, chopped
- ½ medium onion, chopped
- 1 tbsp. fresh parsley, chopped

vinegar, mustard, Herbs de Provence, salt and black pepper and whisk until well combined. Set aside.

2. In a large-sized wok, heat 1 tsp. oil over medium heat and cook the garlic for about 1 minute, stirring continuously.

3. Add in the cooked lentils and cook for about 2 minutes.

4. Remove from heat and transfer into a salad bowl.

5. Stir in the dressing and set aside to cool slightly.

6. Add carrot and onion and stir to combine.

7. Serve with the garnishing of parsley.

Per Serving:

Calories: 181| Fat: 4.3g| Carbs: 26.7g| Fiber: 9.7g| Protein: 10g

---

Chicken Salad

Servings: 04

Prep time: 15 mins

Cooking Time: 18 mins

Ingredients

For Chicken

- 1 tsp. dried thyme
- ½ tsp. garlic powder
- ½ tsp. onion powder
- ¼ tsp. cayenne powder
- ¼ tsp. ground turmeric
- Salt and ground black pepper, as required
- 2 (7-oz.) boneless, skinless chicken breasts, pounded into ¾-inch thickness
- 1 tbsp. olive oil

For Salad

- 5 C. fresh kale, tough ribs removed and chopped
- 1½ C. carrots, peeled and cut into matchsticks
- ¼ C. pine nuts

For Dressing

- 1 small garlic clove, minced

Directions

1. Preheat your oven to 425 °F. Line a baking dish with parchment paper.

2. For chicken: in a bowl, blend together the thyme, spices, salt and black pepper.

3. Drizzle the chicken breasts with oil and then rub with spice mixture generously and drizzle with the oil.

4. Arrange the chicken breasts onto the prepared baking dish.

5. Bake for approximately 16-18 minutes.

6. Remove pan from oven, transfer chicken breasts onto a cutting board for about 5 minutes.

7. For salad: place all ingredients in a salad bowl and mix.

8. For dressing: place all ingredients in another bowl and beat until well combined.

9. Cut each chicken breast into desired-sized slices.

10. Place the salad onto each serving plate and top each with chicken slices.

11. Drizzle with dressing and serve.

- 2 tbsp. fresh lime juice
- 2 tbsp. extra-virgin olive oil
- 1 tsp. maple syrup
- ½ tsp. Dijon mustard
- Salt and ground black pepper, as required

Per Serving:

Calories: 330| Fat: 18.9g| Carbs: 16.5g| Fiber: 2.8g| Protein: 25.3g

Beef & Veggie Soup

Servings: 03
Prep time: 15 mins
Cooking Time: 30 mins

Ingredients

- 2 tbsp. olive oil, divided
- 1 garlic clove, minced
- 8 oz. New York strip steak, trimmed and cubed
- Salt and ground black pepper, as required
- 1 tsp. fresh rosemary, chopped
- ¼ tsp. red pepper flakes, crushed
- ¾ C. fresh shiitake mushrooms, sliced
- ¾ C. fresh kale leaves, tough ribs removed and torn
- 3 C. homemade beef broth
- 1 tbsp. low-sodium soy sauce
- 1 small yellow squash, spiralized with Blade C
- 2 tbsp. scallion, chopped
- ½ tbsp. fresh lime juice

Directions

1. In a Dutch oven, heat 1 tbsp. of the oil over medium heat and sauté the garlic for about 1 minute.
2. Add the beef with salt and black pepper and cook for about 4-5 minutes or until browned.
3. Transfer the beef into a bowl.
4. In the same pan, heat the remaining oil over medium heat and sauté the rosemary and red pepper flakes for about 1 minute.
5. Add the mushrooms and kale and cook for about 2-3 minutes.
6. Add the cooked beef and broth and bring to a boil.
7. Adjust the heat to low and simmer for about 10-15 minutes
8. Add the soy sauce and squash noodles and simmer for about 5 minutes more.
9. Stir in scallion, lemon juice, salt and black pepper and remove from heat.
10. Serve hot.

Per Serving:

Calories: 341| Fat: 22.3g| Carbs: 10.3g| Fiber: 1.8g| Protein: 27.1g

Pasta & Beans Soup

Servings: 06
Prep time: 15 mins
Cooking Time: 45 mins

Ingredients

- 2 tbsp. olive oil
- 1 onion, chopped
- 2 celery stalks, chopped
- Salt and ground black pepper, as required
- 3 C. butternut squash, peeled and cubed
- 4 garlic cloves, minced
- 1 tsp. dried oregano
- 4 C. tomatoes, finely chopped
- 6 C. homemade vegetable broth
- 3 C. Swiss chard, chopped
- 24 oz. cooked cannellini beans
- ½ lb. cooked whole-wheat pasta
- ¼ C. fresh parsley, minced

Directions

1. In a Dutch oven, heat the olive oil over medium-high heat and sauté the onions, celery, salt and black pepper for about 5-7 minutes.
2. Stir in the butternut squash, garlic, and oregano and cook for about 6-8 minutes, stirring occasionally.
3. Add in the tomatoes and broth and bring to a boil.
4. Add the Swiss chard and mix well.
5. Adjust the heat to low and simmer for about 10-15 minutes.
6. Add in the beans and cooked pasta and cook for about 8-10 minutes.
7. Stir in the salt and black pepper and remove from heat.
8. Serve hot with the garnishing of parsley.

Per Serving:
Calories: 300| Fat: 7.3g| Carbs: 46g| Fiber: 11.3g| Protein: 15.3g

Chicken With Veggies

Servings: 04
Prep time: 15 mins
Cooking Time: 1¼ hrs

Ingredients

- 3 tbsp. olive oil, divided
- 6 (6-oz.) bone-in, skinless chicken thighs
- Salt and ground black pepper, as required
- 1 medium onion, chopped

Directions

1. Season the chicken thighs with salt and black pepper evenly.
2. In a heavy-bottomed cast-iron wok, heat 2 tbsp. of oil over medium-high heat and sear the chicken thighs for about 3-4 minutes per side.
3. With a slotted spoon, transfer the chicken thighs onto a

- 2 tbsp. garlic, minced
- 1 large carrot, peeled and sliced
- 2 small red bell peppers, seeded and chopped
- 10 oz. fresh mushrooms, sliced
- 4 tbsp. fresh basil, chopped
- 1 tsp. dried oregano
- ½ C. black olives, pitted
- ¾ C. homemade chicken broth
- 3 C. tomatoes, chopped finely

plate.

4. In the same wok, heat the remaining oil over medium heat and sauté the onion and garlic for about 4-5 minutes.

5. Add the carrot, bell peppers, mushrooms and herbs and cook for about 5 minutes.

6. Add the wine and cook for about 2-3 minutes, scraping up the browned bits from the bottom of the wok.

7. Add the tomatoes, tomato paste, salt and black pepper and stir to combine.

8. Add the chicken thighs and stir to combine.

9. Reduce heat to low and simmer, covered for about 40 minutes, stirring occasionally.

10. Stir in the olives and simmer for about 10 minutes.

11. Serve immediately.

Per Serving:
Calories: 488| Fat: 21.5g| Carbs: 17.4g| Fiber: 4.5g | Protein: 53.5g

Pasta & Beans Soup

Servings: 06
Prep time: 15 mins
Cooking Time: 45 mins

Ingredients

- 2 tbsp. olive oil
- 1 onion, chopped
- 2 celery stalks, chopped
- Salt and ground black pepper, as required
- 3 C. butternut squash, peeled and cubed
- 4 garlic cloves, minced
- 1 tsp. dried oregano
- 4 C. tomatoes, finely chopped
- 6 C. homemade vegetable broth
- 3 C. Swiss chard, chopped
- 24 oz. cooked cannellini beans

Directions

1. In a Dutch oven, heat the olive oil over medium-high heat and sauté the onions, celery, salt and black pepper for about 5-7 minutes.

2. Stir in the butternut squash, garlic, and oregano and cook for about 6-8 minutes, stirring occasionally.

3. Add in the tomatoes and broth and bring to a boil.

4. Add the Swiss chard and mix well.

5. Adjust the heat to low and simmer for about 10-15 minutes.

6. Add in the beans and cooked pasta and cook for about 8-10 minutes.

7. Stir in the salt and black pepper and remove from heat.

8. Serve hot with the garnishing of parsley.

- ½ lb. cooked whole-wheat pasta
- ¼ C. fresh parsley, minced

Per Serving:

Calories: 300| Fat: 7.3g| Carbs: 46g| Fiber: 11.3g| Protein: 15.3g

Barley & Beans Soup

Servings: 04
Prep time: 15 mins
Cooking Time: 40ins

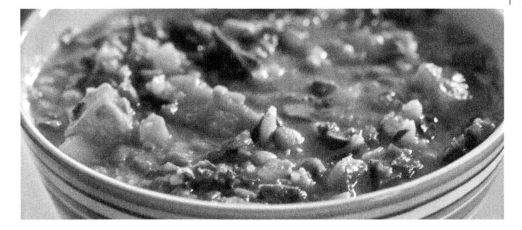

Ingredients

- 1 tbsp. olive oil
- 1 white onion, chopped
- 2 celery stalks, chopped
- 1 large carrot, peeled and chopped
- 2 tbsp. fresh rosemary, chopped
- 2 garlic cloves, minced
- 4 C. fresh tomatoes, chopped
- 4 C. homemade vegetable broth
- 1 C. pearl barley
- 2 C. cooked white beans
- 2 tbsp. fresh lemon juice
- 4 tbsp. fresh parsley leaves, chopped

Directions

1. In a large-sized soup pan, heat the oil over medium heat and sauté the onion, celery and carrot for about 4-5 minutes.
2. Add the garlic and rosemary and sauté for about 1 minute.
3. Add the tomatoes and cook for 3-4 minutes, crushing with the back of a spoon.
4. Add the barley and broth and bring to a boil.
5. Adjust the heat to low and simmer, covered for about 20-25 minutes.
6. Stir in the beans and lemon juice and simmer for about 5 minutes more.
7. Garnish with parsley and serve hot.

Per Serving:

Calories: 392| Fat: 5.6g| Carbs: 71g| Fiber: 18.9g| Protein: 16.1g

Chicken & Kale Stew

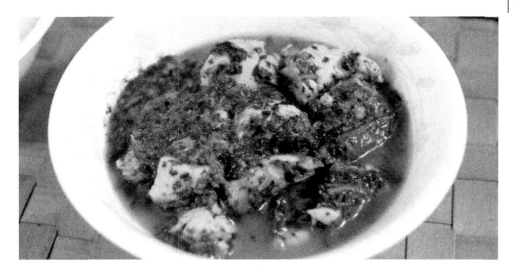

Ingredients

- 2 tbsp. olive oil
- 1 yellow onion, chopped
- 1 tbsp. garlic, minced
- 1 tbsp. fresh ginger, minced
- 1 tsp. ground turmeric
- 1 tsp. ground cumin
- 1 tsp. ground coriander
- 1 tsp. paprika
- 4 (6-oz.) boneless, skinless chicken thighs, trimmed and cut into 1-inch pieces
- 4 tomatoes, chopped
- 12 oz. unsweetened coconut milk
- ¼ C. homemade chicken broth
- Salt and ground black pepper, as required
- 6 C. fresh kale, tough ribs removed and chopped
- 2 tbsp. fresh lemon juice

Directions

1. Heat oil in a large-sized heavy-bottomed pan over medium heat and sauté the onion for about 3-4 minutes.
2. Add the ginger, garlic, and spices, and sauté for about 1 minute.
3. Add the chicken and cook for about 4-5 minutes.
4. Add the tomatoes, coconut milk, broth, salt, and black pepper, and bring to a gentle simmer.
5. Now, adjust the heat to low and simmer, covered for about 10-15 minutes.
6. Stir in the kale and cook for about 4-5 minutes.
7. Add in lemon juice and remove from heat.
8. Serve hot.

Per Serving:

Calories: 248| Fat: 10.7g| Carbs: 14.2g| Fiber: 3g| Protein: 25.6g

Braised Chicken Thighs

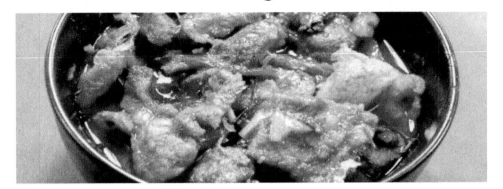

Servings: 06

Prep time: 15 mins

Cooking Time: 55 mins

Ingredients

- 6 (8-oz.) bone-in chicken thighs
- Salt and ground black pepper, as required
- 2 tbsp. olive oil
- ½ of onion, sliced
- 3 C. homemade chicken broth
- ½ tsp. ground turmeric
- 8 sprigs fresh dill
- 2 tbsp. fresh lemon juice
- ½ tbsp. fresh dill, chopped

Directions

1. Sprinkle the chicken thighs with salt and black pepper.
2. In a large-sized non-stick wok, heat the olive oil over high heat.
3. Place the chicken thighs in wok, skin side down and cook for about 3-4 minutes.
4. With a slotted spoon, transfer the thighs onto a plate.
5. In the same wok, add onion over medium heat and sauté for about 4-5 minutes.
6. Return the thighs in wok, skin side up with broth, turmeric, salt and black pepper.
7. Place the dill sprigs and over thighs and bring to a boil.
8. Adjust the heat to medium-low and simmer, covered for about 40-45 minutes, coating the thighs with cooking liquid.
9. Discard the thyme sprigs and stir in the lemon juice.
10. Serve hot with the topping of chopped dill.

Per Serving:

Calories: 499| Fat: 22.3g| Carbs: 2.3g| Fiber: 0.4g | Protein: 68.4g

Veggie Stew

Servings: 04

Prep time: 15 mins

Cooking Time: 45 mins

Ingredients

- 1 tbsp. olive oil
- 14 oz. fresh mushrooms, sliced
- 1 small onion, chopped
- 4 garlic cloves, minced
- 1 tsp. fresh thyme, chopped
- 1 tsp. onion powder
- ¼ tsp. red pepper flakes
- Salt, as required
- 2 C. homemade vegetable broth
- 1 C. carrots, chopped
- 1 C. celery, chopped
- 1 tbsp. almond flour
- 2 tbsp. water
- ¼ C. parsley, chopped

Directions

1. In a deep non-stick wok, heat the oil over medium heat and sauté the mushrooms, onion, and garlic for about 4-5 minutes.
2. Add in the thyme, onion powder, red pepper flakes and salt and cook for about 1 minute, stirring frequently.
3. Add in the broth, carrots and celery and bring to a boil.
4. Adjust the heat to medium-low and cook, covered for about 30 minutes.
5. Meanwhile, for flour slurry: in a small-sized bowl, dissolve the almond flour into water.
6. In the pan, add the flour slurry, stirring continuously.
7. Cook for about 1-2 minutes, stirring continuously.
8. Stir in the parsley and serve hot.

Per Serving:

Calories: 112| Fat: 5.5g| Carbs: 11.1g| Fiber: 3g| Protein: 6.9g

Chickpeas & Spinach Stew

Servings: 04

Prep time: 15 mins

Cooking Time: 30 mins

Ingredients

- 1 tbsp. olive oil
- 1 medium onion, chopped
- 2 C. carrots, peeled and chopped
- 2 garlic cloves, minced
- 1 tsp. red pepper flakes
- 2 large tomatoes, peeled,

Directions

1. In a large-sized pan, heat oil over medium heat and sauté the onion and carrot for about 6 minutes.
2. Stir in the garlic and red pepper flakes and sauté for about 1 minute.
3. Add the tomatoes and cook for about 2-3 minutes.
4. Add the broth and bring to a boil.

seeded and chopped finely

- 2 C. homemade vegetable broth
- 2 C. cooked chickpeas
- 2 C. fresh spinach, chopped
- 1 tbsp. fresh lemon juice
- Salt and ground black pepper, as required

5. Adjust the heat to low and simmer for about 10 minutes.

6. Stir in the chickpeas and simmer for about 5 minutes.

7. Stir in the spinach and simmer for 3-4 minutes more.

8. Stir in the lemon juice and seasoning and remove from heat.

9. Serve hot.

Per Serving:

Calories: 217| Fat: 6.6g| Carbs: 31.4g| Fiber: 9.5g| Protein: 10.6g

Chicken With Capers Sauce

Servings: 04
Prep time: 15 mins
Cooking Time: 10 mins

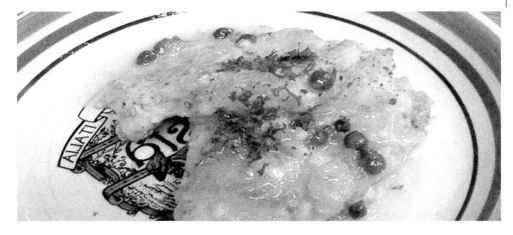

Ingredients

- ¼ C. almond flour
- ¼ C. low-fat Parmesan cheese, grated
- ¼ tsp. red pepper flakes
- Salt and ground black pepper, as required
- 4 (4-oz.) boneless chicken cutlets
- 3 tbsp. olive oil, divided
- 1 shallot, peeled and finely

Directions

1. In a large-sized shallow bowl, add the almond flour, Parmesan cheese, red pepper flakes, salt and black pepper and mix well.

2. Coat the chicken with the flour mixture evenly.

3. In a wok, heat half of the oil over medium heat and cook the chicken pieces for about 3-5 minutes per side.

4. With a slotted spoon, transfer the chicken pieces onto a plate and cover with a piece of foil to keep warm.

5. In the same wok, heat remaining oil over medium heat

- diced
- 2 garlic cloves, minced
- ¼ C. capers, drained
- ¾ C. homemade chicken broth
- ¼ C. fresh lemon juice

and sauté the shallot and garlic for about 3 minutes.

6. Stir in the capers, broth and lemon juice and cook for about 5 minutes.

7. Remove from heat and pour over the chicken breasts.

8. Serve immediately.

Per Serving:
Calories: 259| Fat: 11.9g| Carbs: 7.4g| Fiber: 0.6g | Protein: 30.3g

---

Tuna With Olives

Servings: 04
Prep time: 15 mins
Cooking Time: 10 mins

Ingredients

- Olive oil cooking spray
- 4 (6-oz.) (1-inch thick) tuna steaks
- 2 tbsp. olive oil, divided
- Salt and ground black pepper, as required
- 2 garlic cloves, minced
- 1 C. fresh tomatoes, chopped
- 1 C. homemade chicken broth
- 2/3 C. green olives, pitted and sliced
- ¼ C. capers, drained
- 2 tbsp. fresh thyme, chopped
- 1½ tbsp. fresh lemon zest, grated
- 2 tbsp. fresh lemon juice
- 3 tbsp. fresh parsley, chopped

Directions

1. Preheat the grill to high heat. Grease the grill grate with cooking spray.

2. Coat the tuna steaks with 1 tbsp. of the oil and sprinkle with salt and black pepper.

3. Set aside for about 5 minutes.

4. For sauce: in a small-sized wok, heat the remaining oil over medium heat and sauté the garlic for about 1 minute.

5. Add the tomatoes and cook for about 2 minutes.

6. Stir in the wine and bring to a boil.

7. Add the remaining ingredients except for parsley and cook, uncovered for about 5 minutes.

8. Stir in the parsley, salt and black pepper and remove from heat.

9. Meanwhile, place the tuna steaks over direct heat and cook for about 1-2 minutes per side.

10. Serve the tuna steaks hot with the topping of sauce.

Per Serving:

Calories: 468| Fat: 10.7g| Carbs: 7.3g| Fiber: 2.3g | Protein: 52.1g

---

Stuffed Steak

Servings: 06
Prep time: 15 mins
Cooking Time: 35 mins

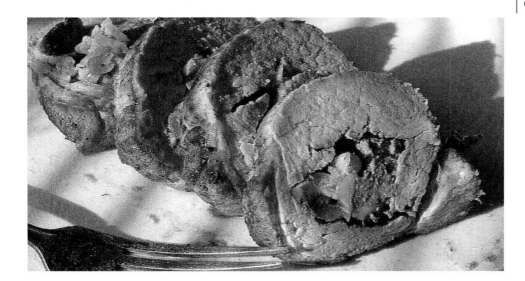

Ingredients

- 2 tbsp. dried oregano leaves
- 1/3 C. fresh lemon juice
- 2 tbsp. olive oil
- 1 (2-lb.) beef flank steak, trimmed and pounded into ½-inch thickness
- 1/3 C. olive tapenade
- 1 C. frozen chopped spinach, thawed and squeezed
- ¼ C. low-fat feta cheese, crumbled
- Salt, as required

Directions

1. In a large-sized baking dish, add the oregano, lemon juice and oil and mix well.
2. Add the steak and coat with the marinade generously.
3. Refrigerate to marinate for about 4 hours, flipping occasionally.
4. Preheat your oven to 425 °F. Line a shallow baking dish with parchment paper.
5. Remove the steak from the baking dish.
6. Arrange the steak onto a cutting board.
7. Place the tapenade onto the steak evenly and top with the spinach, followed by the feta cheese.
8. Carefully roll the steak tightly to form a log.
9. With 6 kitchen string pieces, tie the log at 6 places.
10. Carefully cut the log between strings into 6 equal pieces, leaving the string in place.

11. Arrange the log pieces onto the prepared baking dish, cut-side up.

12. Bake for approximately 25-35 minutes.

13. Remove from oven and set aside for about 5 minutes before serving.

Per Serving:

Calories: 395| Fat: 18.2g| Carbs: 7.3g| Fiber: 2.2g | Protein: 48.8g

Braised Beef

Servings: 12

Prep time: 15 mins

Cooking Time: 1 hrs 55 mins

Ingredients

- ¼ C. olive oil
- 3 lb. boneless beef chuck roast, trimmed and cut into 1½-inch cubes
- 3 celery stalks, chopped
- 2 onions, chopped
- 4 garlic cloves, minced
- 6-8 C. tomatoes, finely chopped
- 1½ C. homemade chicken broth
- ½ C. fresh parsley, chopped
- 1 tsp. dried oregano
- Salt and ground black pepper, as required

Directions

1. In a large-sized pan, heat the oil over medium-high heat and sear the beef cubes for about 4-5 minutes.

2. Add the celery, onions and garlic and cook for about 5 minutes, stirring frequently.

3. Stir in the remaining ingredients and bring to a boil.

4. Reduce heat to low and simmer, covered for about 1½-1¾ hours or until desired doneness of beef.

5. Serve hot.

Per Serving:

Calories: 278| Fat: 11.7g| Carbs: 6g| Fiber: 1.7g| Protein: 36.2g

Parmesan Tilapia

Servings: 04
Prep time: 10 mins
Cooking Time: 11 mins

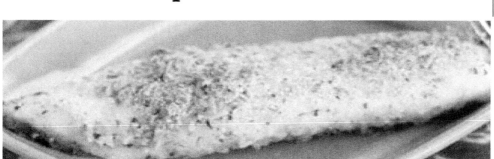

Ingredients

- Olive oil cooking spray
- 4 (6-oz.) tilapia fillets
- Salt and ground black pepper, as required
- ½ C. low-fat Parmesan cheese, grated
-

Directions

1. Preheat the broiler of oven. Line a baking sheet with a piece of foil and then spray it with cooking spray.
2. Season the tilapia fillets with salt and black pepper lightly.
3. Arrange the tilapia fillets onto the prepared baking sheet in a single layer and top each with Parmesan cheese evenly.
4. Broil for about 10-11 minutes.
5. Remove from oven and serve hot.

Per Serving:

Calories: 173| Fat: 4g| Carbs: 0.2g| Fiber: 0g| Protein: 34.1g

Maple Glazed Salmon

Servings: 06
Prep time: 10 mins
Cooking Time: 18 mins

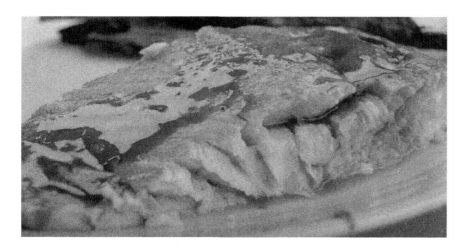

Ingredients

- 1 tbsp. red pepper flakes, crushed
- 1/8 tsp. ground cinnamon
- Ground black pepper, as required
- 6 (6-oz.) fresh salmon fillets
- 2 tbsp. fresh lemon juice
- 4 tsp. extra-virgin olive oil, divided
- ¼ C. pure maple syrup
- ¼ C. low-sodium soy sauce
- ¼ C. scallion, chopped

Directions

1. In a small-sized bowl, blend together all spices and set aside.
2. In a large-sized bowl, place salmon fillets, lemon juice, 2 tsp. of oil and spice mixture and toss to coat well.
3. Cover and refrigerate for at least 2 hours.
4. In a small-sized cast-iron wok, blend together maple syrup and soy sauce over medium heat and cook for about 7-10 minutes, stirring occasionally.
5. Meanwhile, in a large-sized cast-iron wok, heat the remaining oil over high heat.
6. Place the salmon fillets, flesh side down and cook for about 4 minutes.
7. Carefully flip the side and add maple syrup glaze.
8. Cook for about 4 minutes more.
9. Transfer the fillets onto serving plates.
10. Top with the glaze from pan and serve with the garnishing of the scallion.

Per Serving:

Calories: 297| Fat: 13.8g| Carbs: 10.6g| Fiber: 0.5g| Protein: 33.9g

Stuffed Salmon

Servings: 04
Prep time: 15 mins
Cooking Time: 16 mins

Ingredients

- 4 C. fresh spinach, chopped
- ½ C. artichoke hearts, drained and chopped
- ½ C. oil-packed sun-dried tomatoes, drained and chopped
- ¼ C. low-fat feta cheese, crumbled
- 4 (8-oz.) salmon fillets
- Pinch of garlic powder
- Salt and ground black pepper, as required

Directions

1. In a saucepan of lightly salted boiling water, cook the spinach for about 40 seconds.
2. In a colander, drain the spinach and immediately immerse in a bowl of ice water.
3. Again, drain the spinach completely and transfer into a bowl.
4. In the bowl of spinach, add the artichokes, sun-dried tomatoes and feta cheese and mix well.
5. With a sharp knife, make a horizontal cut in the center of each salmon fillet. (Do not cut all the way through).
6. Season each salmon fillet with garlic powder, salt, and

black pepper.

7. Stuff each salmon pocket with spinach mixture evenly.
8. Heat a cast-iron wok over medium heat.
9. In the wok, place the salmon fillets, skin-sides down and cook for about 5 minutes.
10. Carefully flip the fillets and cook for about 5 minutes.
11. Again, flip the fillets and cook for about 5 minutes.
12. Serve hot.

Per Serving:

Calories: 345| Fat: 16.3g| Carbs: 4.4g| Fiber: 1.9g| Protein: 47.1g

---

Barley & Veggie Pilaf

Servings: 04
Prep time: 15 mins
Cooking Time: 1 hrs 5 mins

Ingredients

- ½ C. pearl barley
- 1 C. homemade vegetable broth
- 2 tbsp. olive oil, divided
- 2 garlic cloves, minced
- ½ C. white onion, chopped
- ½ C. green olives, sliced
- ½ C. green bell pepper, seeded and chopped
- ½ C. red bell pepper, seeded and chopped
- 2 tbsp. fresh cilantro, chopped
- 2 tbsp. fresh mint leaves, chopped
- 1 tbsp. low-sodium soy sauce

Directions

1. In a saucepan, add the barley and broth over medium-high heat and cook until boiling.
2. Immediately, Adjust the heat to low and simmer, covered for about 45 minutes or until all the liquid is evaporated.
3. In a large-sized wok, heat 1 tbsp. of the oil over medium-high heat and sauté the garlic for about 30 seconds.
4. Stir in the cooked barley and cook for about 3 minutes.
5. Remove from heat and set aside.
6. In another wok, heat the remaining oil over medium heat and sauté the onion for about 7 minutes.
7. Add the olives and bell pepper and stir fry for about 3 minutes.
8. Stir in remaining ingredients except and cook for about 3 minutes.
9. Stir in the barley mixture and cook for about 3 minutes.
10. Serve hot with the garnishing of walnuts.

Per Serving:

Calories: 204| Fat: 10.1g| Carbs: 25.3g| Fiber: 4.9g| Protein: 4.8g

Lentils With Kale

Servings: 06

Prep time: 15 mins

Cooking Time: 20 mins

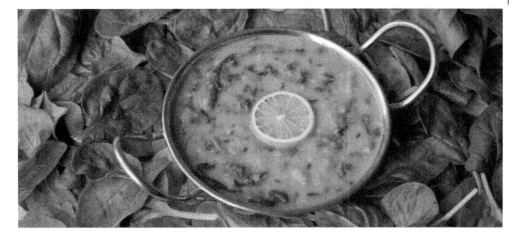

Ingredients

- 1½ C. red lentils, rinsed
- 1½ C. homemade vegetable broth
- 1½ tbsp. olive oil
- ½ C. onion, chopped
- 1 tsp. fresh ginger, minced
- 2 garlic cloves, minced
- 1½ C. tomato, chopped
- 6 C. fresh kale, tough ends removed and chopped
- Salt and ground black pepper, as required

Directions

1. In a saucepan, add the broth and lentils over medium-high heat and bring to a boil.
2. Adjust the heat to and simmer, covered for about 20 minutes or until almost all the liquid is absorbed.
3. Remove from heat and set aside covered.
4. Meanwhile, in a large-sized wok, heat oil over medium heat and sauté the onion for about 5-6 minutes.
5. Add the ginger and garlic and sauté for about 1 minute.
6. Add tomatoes and kale and cook for about 4-5 minutes.
7. Stir in the lentils, salt and black pepper and remove from heat.
8. Serve hot.

Per Serving:

Calories: 257| Fat: 4.5g| Carbs: 39.3g| Fiber: 16.5g| Protein: 16.2g

SNACKS

Recipes

By: Lara Rush

Spiced Almonds

Servings: 05
Prep time: 5 mins
Cooking Time: 10 mins

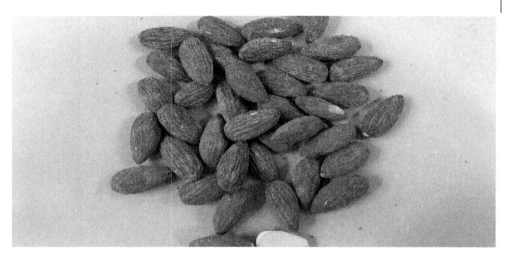

Ingredients

- 1 C. whole almonds
- ½ tsp. ground cinnamon
- ¼ tsp. ground cumin
- Salt and ground black pepper 2 tbsp. olive oil

Directions

1. Preheat your oven to 350 °F.
2. Line a baking dish with parchment paper.
3. Add all ingredients in a bowl and toss to coat well.
4. Spread the almonds into the prepared baking dish in a single layer.
5. Roast for approximately 10 minutes, flipping twice.
6. Remove from oven and let the almonds cool completely before serving..

Per Serving:

Calories: 198| Fat: 18.9g| Carbs: 5.3g| Fiber: 3.1g| Protein: 4g

---

Glazed Cashews

Servings: 08
Prep time: 10 mins
Cooking Time: 12 mins

Ingredients

- 1 tbsp. maple syrup
- 1 tbsp. coconut oil, melted
- 2 tbsp. Erythritol
- ½ tsp. salt

Directions

1. Preheat your oven to 325°F. Line a baking sheet with parchment paper.
2. In a large-sized bowl, add the maple syrup, coconut oil, Erythritol and salt and mix until the Erythritol is

- 2 C. raw cashews

  dissolved.

  3. Add the cashews and toss to coat well.
  4. Place the cashews onto the prepared baking sheet and spread in an even layer.
  5. Roast for about 10-12 minutes, stirring after every 8 minutes.
  6. Remove from oven and let the cashews cool for 10-12 minutes before serving.

Per Serving:

Calories: 211| Fat: 15.5g| Carbs: 10.7g| Fiber: 7g| Protein: 5g

---

Salted Edamame

Servings: 08
Prep time: 10 mins
Cooking Time: 20 mins

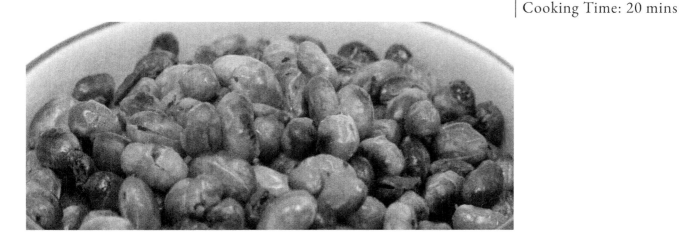

Ingredients

- 2 C. frozen shelled edamame, thawed
- 2 tsp. olive oil
- 1 tsp. salt

Directions

1. Preheat your oven to 450 °F.
2. In a bowl, add all ingredients and toss to coat well.
3. Place the edamame onto the prepared baking sheet and spread in an even layer.
4. Roast for about 15-20 minutes, stirring once halfway through.
5. Remove from oven and let the edamame cool completely before serving.

Per Serving:

Calories: 104| Fat: 5.5g| Carbs: 7.1g| Fiber: 2.7g| Protein: 8.3g

Hummus & Oat Bites

Servings: 08
Prep time: 15 mins

Ingredients

- 2 C. gluten-free old-fashioned oats
- 1 C. hummus
- 1 tbsp. olive oil
- ¼ C. roasted chickpeas
- ¼ C. pumpkin seeds
- ¼ C. sunflower seeds
- ¼ tsp. salt
- ¼ tsp. ground black pepper
- ¼ tsp. red pepper flakes
- 1 tbsp. nutritional yeast

Directions

1. In a large-sized bowl, add all ingredients and mix until well combined.
2. Make small equal-sized balls from the mixture.
3. Serve immediately.

Per Serving:

Calories: 187| Fat: 9.1g| Carbs: 21.4g| Fiber: 4.9g| Protein: 7.3g

---

Brownie Bites

Servings: 10
Prep time: 15 mins

Ingredients

- ¾ C. blanched almond flour
- ¾ C. cacao powder
- 2 tbsp. ground flaxseeds
- ½ C. unsweetened dark chocolate chips
- ¾ C. creamy almond butter, melted
- ¼ C. maple syrup
- 1 tsp. organic vanilla extract

Directions

1. In a large-sized bowl, blend together the almond flour, cocoa powder, flaxseeds and chocolate chips.
2. Add the almond butter, maple syrup and vanilla extract and gently stir to combine.
3. Using a sturdy spatula, stir and fold together until well incorporated.
4. With your hands, make equal-sized balls from mixture.
5. Arrange the balls onto a parchment paper-lined baking sheet in a single layer.
6. Refrigerate to set for about 15 minutes before serving.

Per Serving:

Calories: 182| Fat: 12.7g| Carbs: 14g| Fiber: 4.8g| Protein: 5.1g

Fruity Oat Bites

Servings: 10
Prep time: 15 mins

Ingredients

- 1 ripe banana, peeled
- ¼ C. maple syrup
- ¼ C. sunflower seed butter, melted
- 1½ C. gluten-free quick oats
- ¾ C. gluten-free rolled oats
- 1/3 C. unsweetened protein powder
- 2 tsp. ground flaxseeds
- 1 tsp. vanilla extract
- 1/3 C. dried unsweetened cranberries

Directions

1. In a large-sized bowl, add the banana and with a fork, mash it.
2. Add the maple syrup and sunflower seed butter and mix until smooth.
3. Add the oats, protein powder, flaxseeds and vanilla extract and mix until well combined.
4. Gently fold in the cranberries.
5. With your hands, make equal-sized balls from mixture.
6. Arrange the balls onto a parchment paper-lined baking sheet in a single layer.
7. Refrigerate to set for about 15 minutes before serving.

Per Serving:

Calories: 176| Fat: 4.9g| Carbs: 24.2g| Fiber: 2.8g| Protein: 8.9g

Chocolate Oat Bites

Servings: 12
Prep time: 15 mins

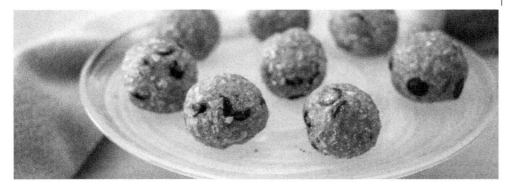

Ingredients

- 2/3 C. creamy peanut butter
- 1 C. gluten-free old-

Directions

1. In a bowl, place all the ingredients and mx until well combined.
2. Refrigerate for about 20-30 minutes.

fashioned oats
- ½ C. unsweetened dark chocolate chips
- ½ C. ground flaxseeds
- 2 tbsp. maple syrup

3. With your hands, make equal-sized balls from mixture.
4. Arrange the balls onto a parchment paper-lined baking sheet in a single layer.
5. Refrigerate to set for about 15 minutes before serving.

Per Serving:

Calories: 209| Fat: 14.5g| Carbs: 13.6g| Fiber: 4.1g| Protein: 6.6g

Cranberry Bars

Servings: 16
Prep time: 20 mins
Cooking Time: 35 mins

Ingredients

- Olive oil cooking spray
- 1 C. fresh cranberries, chopped finely
- 2 tsp. powdered Erythritol
- ¼ C. almond flour
- ¼ C. coconut flour
- ¼ C. golden flaxseed meal
- 1 tsp. baking powder
- Pinch of salt
- 6 tbsp. coconut oil, softened
- 1/3 C. granulated Erythritol
- 2 eggs
- 1 tsp. organic vanilla extract

Directions

1. Preheat your oven to 350 ºF. Grease an 8x8-inch baking dish with cooking spray.
2. In a small-sized bowl, add the cranberries and powdered Erythritol and toss to coat well.
3. In a bowl, add flours, flaxseed meal, baking powder, and salt and mix well.
4. In a separate large-sized bowl, add almond butter and granulated Erythritol and mix well.
5. Add 1 egg and whisk well.
6. Repeat with the remaining egg.
7. Add vanilla extract and mix well.
8. Slowly add flour mixture and mix until just blended.
9. Fold in cranberries.
10. Place the bar mixture into the prepared baking dish and with the back of a spoon, smooth the top surface.
11. Bake for approximately 30-35 minutes.
12. Remove the baking dish of bars from oven and place onto a wire rack to cool completely.
13. Cut into equal-sized bars and serve.

Per Serving:

Calories: 90| Fat: 5.4g| Carbs: 5.5g| Fiber: 1.4g| Protein: 1.7g

Nuts & Seeds Bars

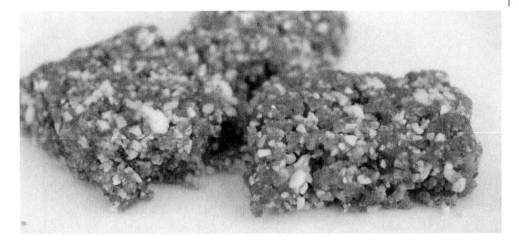

Ingredients

- Olive oil cooking spray
- 1½ C. gluten-free rolled oats
- ½ C. almonds, chopped roughly
- ½ C. cashews, chopped roughly
- ½ C. mini unsweetened dark chocolate chips
- 1/3 C. pumpkin seeds
- ¼ C. sesame seeds
- ¼ C. sunflower seeds
- ¼ C. flaxseed meal
- 2 tbsp. chia seeds
- 1 tsp. ground cinnamon
- ½ C. maple syrup
- 1 C. almond butter, softened

Directions

1. Line an 8x8-inch baking dish with parchment paper and then grease it with cooking spray.
2. In a large-sized bowl, add oats, nuts, chocolate chips, seeds and cinnamon and mix well.
3. Add in the maple syrup and stir to combine.
4. Add the almond butter and mix until well combined.
5. Place oat mixture into the prepared baking dish evenly and with the back of a spatula, smooth the top surface by pressing in the bottom.
6. Refrigerate for about 6-8 hours or until set completely.
7. Cut into desired-sized bars and serve.

Per Serving:

Calories: 282| Fat: 17.4g| Carbs: 25.6g| Fiber: 5.3g| Protein: 7.9g

Carrot Cookies

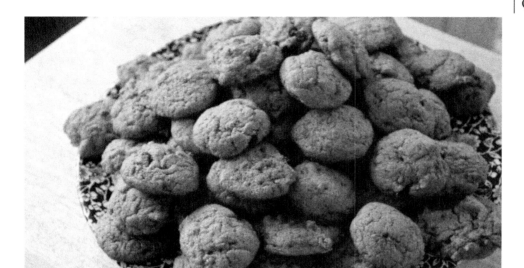

Ingredients

- ¾ C. almond flour
- ¼ C. coconut flour
- ¼ tsp. baking soda
- ¼ tsp. salt
- 1 large organic egg
- ¾ C. Erythritol
- 4 tbsp. coconut oil, melted
- 1 tsp. organic vanilla extract
- 1/3 C. walnuts, chopped
- ¼ C. carrots, peeled, shredded and chopped

Directions

1. Preheat your oven to 350 ºF. Line a large-sized cookie sheet with parchment paper.
2. In a bowl, add the flours, baking soda and salt and mix well.
3. In another large bowl, add the egg, Erythritol, butter and vanilla extract and beat until well combined.
4. Add the flour mixture and mix until a dough forms.
5. Gently fold in the walnuts and carrots.
6. With a 1-inch cookie scooper, scoop 12 cookies onto the prepared cookie sheets in a single layer about 4-inch apart.
7. With your palm, flatten each cookie slightly.
8. Bake for approximately 12-14 minutes or until edges become golden brown.
9. Remove from oven and place onto a wire rack to cool in the pan for about 5-10 minutes.
10. Ten invert the cookies onto the wire rack to cool completely before serving.

Per Serving:

Calories: 105| Fat: 9.8g| Carbs: 2.1g| Fiber: 1.1g| Protein: 3g

Spiced Cookies

Servings: 05
Prep time: 15 mins
Cooking Time: 9 mins

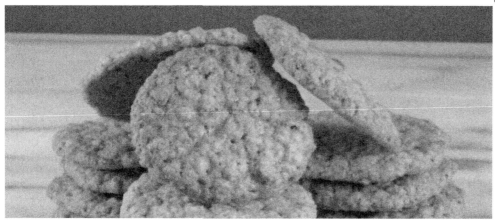

Ingredients

- 1/3 C. coconut flour
- ¼ tsp. whole fennel seeds
- Pinch of ground cinnamon
- Pinch of ground cardamom
- Pinch of sea salt
- Pinch of ground black pepper
- ¼ C. coconut oil, softened
- 2 tbsp. maple syrup
- 1 tsp. organic vanilla extract
- ½ tsp. fresh ginger root, grated finely

Directions

1. Preheat your oven to 360 °F. Line a cookie sheet with parchment paper.
2. In a large-sized bowl, add the flour, fennel seeds, spices, salt, and black pepper and mix well.
3. In another bowl, add the coconut oil, maple syrup, and vanilla extract and beat until well combined.
4. Add the ginger and stir to combine.
5. Add the flour mixture and mix until a smooth dough forms.
6. Make small, equal-sized balls from the mixture.
7. Arrange the balls onto the prepared cookie sheet about 1-inch apart in a single layer and, with your fingers, gently press down each ball to form the cookies.
8. Bake for 9 minutes or until golden brown.
9. Remove from oven and place the cookie sheet onto a wire rack to cool in the pan for about 5 minutes.
10. Carefully invert the cookies onto the wire rack to cool completely before serving..

Per Serving:

Calories: 122| Fat: 11.1g| Carbs: 6.2g| Fiber: 0.4g| Protein: 0.2g

Chickpeas Fries

Servings: 08
Prep time: 20 mins
Cooking Time: 50 mins

Ingredients

- Olive oil cooking spray
- 4 C. water
- 2 C. chickpea flour
- ½ C. green bell pepper, seeded and chopped
- ½ C. onions, chopped
- 1 tbsp. fresh oregano, chopped
- 1 tsp. onion powder
- 1 tsp. cayenne powder
- Sea salt, as required

Directions

1. Grease 2 parchment papers with cooking spray.
2. Line a baking sheet with 1greased parchment paper.
3. In a large-sized pan, add the water and flour over medium heat and beat until well combined.
4. Add the remaining ingredients and cook for about 10 minutes, stirring frequently.
5. Remove from heat and place the mixture onto the prepared baking sheet.
6. With a spatula, smooth the top surface.
7. With another greased parchment paper, cover the surface and with another baking sheet, press tightly.
8. Freeze for about 20 minutes.
9. Preheat your oven to 400 ºF.
10. Lightly grease a baking sheet.
11. Remove the parchment paper from top and cut into desired-sized fries.
12. Arrange the fries onto the prepared baking sheet in a single layer,
13. Bake for approximately 20 minutes.
14. Carefully flip the fries over and bake for approximately 10-15 minutes.
15. Serve warm.

Per Serving:
Calories: 98| Fat: 1.7g| Carbs: 15.3g | Fiber: 3.1g| Protein: 5.4g

---

Brussels Sprout Chips

Servings: 04
Prep time: 15 mins
Cooking Time: 20 mins

Ingredients

- Olive oil cooking spray

Directions

1. Preheat your oven to 400 °F.

- ½ lb. Brussels sprout, sliced thinly
- 4 tbsp. low-fat Parmesan cheese, grated and divided
- 1 tbsp. olive oil
- 1 tsp. garlic powder
- Salt and ground black pepper, as required

2. Lightly grease a large-sized baking sheet with cooking spray.
3. Place the Brussels sprout slices, 2 tbsp. of Parmesan cheese, oil, garlic powder, salt, and black pepper in a large-sized mixing bowl and toss to coat well.
4. Arrange the Brussels sprout slices onto the prepared baking sheet in an even layer.
5. Bake for approximately 18-20 minutes, tossing once halfway through.
6. Remove from oven and transfer the Brussels sprout chips onto a platter.
7. Sprinkle with the remaining cheese and serve.

Per Serving:

Calories: 100| Fat: 6.5g| Carbs: 7.6g| Fiber: 2.9g| Protein: 5.4g

Carrot Hummus

Servings: 08

Prep time: 15 mins

Cooking Time: 30 mins

Ingredients

- 3 carrots, peeled and chopped roughly
- 3 tbsp. extra-virgin olive oil, divided
- 1 tsp. paprika, divided
- Salt, as required
- 1 garlic clove, peeled
- 1 (15-oz.) cooked chickpeas
- 1½ tbsp. tahini
- 2 tbsp. fresh lemon juice
- 6 tbsp. water
- ½ tsp. ground cumin

Directions

1. Preheat your oven to 400 °F.
2. Line a large-sized baking sheet with parchment paper.
3. Place the carrots, 1 tbsp. of oil, ½ tsp. of paprika and a pinch of salt onto the prepared abaking sheet and toss to coat well.
4. Then, spread the carrot pieces in an even layer.
5. Bake for approximately 25 minutes.
6. Place the garlic clove onto the baking sheet with carrot pieces and bake for approximately 10 minutes.
7. Remove the baking sheet of carrot from oven and set aside to cool.
8. In a food processor, add the carrot, garlic and remaining ingredients and pulse until smooth.
9. Serve immediately.

Per Serving:

Calories: 137| Fat: 7.5g| Carbs: 15.3g| Fiber: 3.3g| Protein: 3.4g

Tofu & Veggie Gazpacho

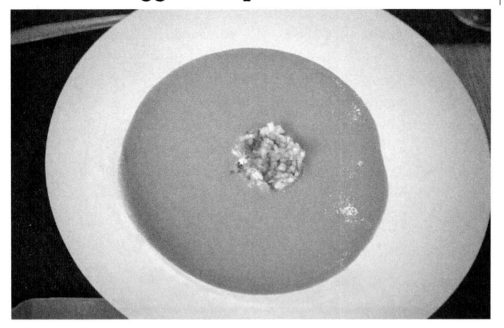

Ingredients

- 7 oz. silken tofu, drained and pressed
- 2 large cucumbers, peeled, seeded and chopped roughly
- ½ of ripe avocado, peeled, pitted and chopped roughly
- 2 scallions, chopped roughly
- 1 C. fresh mint leaves
- 1 C. fresh basil leaves
- 2 tbsp. fresh dill
- 1 garlic clove, peeled
- 2 tbsp. tahini
- 3-4 tbsp. fresh lime juice
- Pinch of paprika
- Salt and ground black pepper, as required
- ¼ C. water

Directions

1. In a food processor, add all ingredients and pulse until smooth.
2. Transfer the gazpacho into a bowl and refrigerate to chill before serving.

Per Serving:
Calories: 226| Fat: 14.3g| Carbs: 19.1g| Fiber: 7g| Protein: 10.1g

DESSERT

Recipes

By: Lara Rush

Baked Pears

Servings: 04
Prep time: 10 mins
Cooking Time: 25 mins

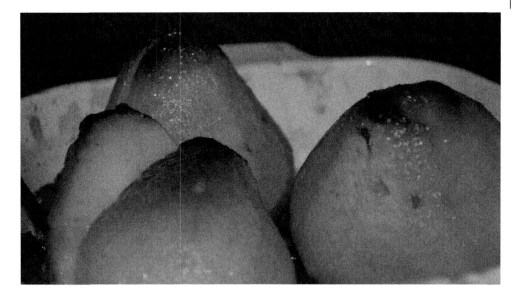

Ingredients

- 4 Anjou pears, halved and cored
- ¼ tsp. ground cinnamon
- ½ C. maple syrup
- 1 tsp. organic vanilla extract

Directions

1. Preheat your oven to 375 °F. Line a baking sheet with parchment paper.
2. Carefully cut a small-sized sliver off the underside of each pear half.
3. Arrange the pear halves onto the prepared baking sheet, cut side upwards and sprinkle with cinnamon.
4. In a small-sized bowl, add the maple syrup and vanilla extract and beat well.
5. Reserve about 2 tbsp. of the maple syrup mixture.
6. Place the remaining maple syrup mixture over the pears and bake for approximately 25 minutes or until lightly browned.
7. Remove from oven and immediately drizzle with the reserved maple syrup mixture.
8. Serve warm.

Per Serving:

Calories: 227| Fat: 0.4g| Carbs: 58.5g| Fiber: 6.6g| Protein: 0.8g

Coffee Granita

Servings: 08
Prep time: 10 mins

Ingredients

- 4 C. hot brewed extra strong coffee
- 2 tsp. ground cinnamon
- ½ C. Erythritol
- ¼ C. coconut cream

Directions

1. In a large-sized bowl, add coffee, cinnamon and Erythritol and stir until Erythritol is completely dissolved.
2. Add coconut cream and beat until well combined.
3. Refrigerate for about 30 minutes.
4. Remove from refrigerator and transfer the mixture into a shallow baking dish.
5. Freeze for about 3 hours, scraping after every 30 minutes with the help of a fork.

Per Serving:

Calories: 20| Fat: 1.8g| Carbs: 0.9g| Fiber: 0.5g| Protein: 0.3g

---

Minty Coconut Mousse

Servings: 04
Prep time: 15 mins

Ingredients

- 1½ C. raw coconut meat, chopped
- 1 tbsp. fresh mint leaves
- 1 tbsp. chia seeds
- 1¼ C. unsweetened almond milk
- 10-12 drops liquid stevia
- ¼ C. almond butter
- 1 tsp. organic vanilla extract

Directions

1. In a blender, add all ingredients except the raspberries and pulse until creamy and smooth.
2. Transfer into serving bowls and refrigerate to chill before serving.

Per Serving:

Calories: 151| Fat: 13.6g| Carbs: 7.1g| Fiber: 4.2g| Protein: 2.4g

Spinach Sorbet

Servings: 04
Prep time: 15 mins

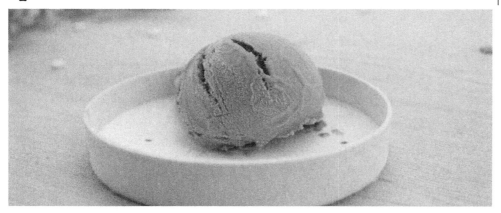

Ingredients

- 3 C. fresh spinach, torn
- 1 tbsp. fresh basil leaves
- ½ of avocado, peeled, pitted and chopped
- ¾ C. unsweetened almond milk
- 20 drops liquid stevia
- 1 tsp. almonds, chopped very finely
- 1 tsp. organic vanilla extract
- 1 C. ice cubes

Directions

1. Transfer into an ice cream maker and process according to manufacturer's directions.
2. Transfer into an airtight container and freeze for at least 4-5 hours before serving.

Per Serving:

Calories: 166| Fat: 16g| Carbs: 5.7g| Fiber: 3.2g| Protein: 2.3g

---

Almond Jelly

Servings: 04
Prep time: 10 mins

Ingredients

- 1 2/3 C. boiling water
- 2 (¼-oz.) envelopes unflavored gelatin
- ½ C. granulated Erythritol
- 4 tsp. organic almond extract

Directions

1. In a bowl, add the boiling water and gelatin and beat vigorously until dissolved.
2. Add Erythritol and gently beat until dissolved.
3. Add almond extract and beat until well combined.
4. Add milk and beat until well combined.
5. Place the mixture into an 8x8-inch baking dish and

- ½ C. cold unsweetened coconut milk

refrigerate to chill for about 2-3 hours or until set completely.

6. Remove from the refrigerator and cut into squares.
7. Serve immediately.

Per Serving:

Calories: 93| Fat: 7.2g| Carbs: 2.2g| Fiber: 0.7g| Protein: 3.7g

---

Crème Brulee

Servings: 04
Prep time: 20 mins
Cooking Time: 6 mins

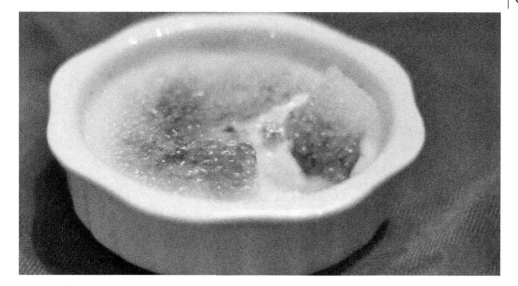

Ingredients

- 1 (13½-oz.) can unsweetened coconut milk
- ¼ C. raw cashews
- ½ C. granulated Erythritol, divided
- 1 tbsp. arrowroot powder
- 1 tsp. nutritional yeast flakes
- 1 tsp. vanilla extract

Directions

1. In a saucepan, add the coconut milk, cashews, ¼ C. of Erythritol and arrowroot powder and stir to combine well.
2. Place the saucepan over medium heat and cook for about 6 minutes, stirring continuously.
3. Remove from heat and set aside to cool slightly.
4. In a high-power blender, add the milk mixture, nutritional yeast flakes, vanilla extract and turmeric and pulse until smooth and creamy.
5. Divide the mixture into 4 ramekins and refrigerate overnight.
6. Just before serving, sprinkle 1 tbsp. of Erythritol on top of each ramekin.

7. Holding a kitchen torch about 4-5-inch from the top, caramelize the Erythritol for about 2 minutes.

8. Set aside for 5 minutes before serving.

Per Serving:

Calories: 82| Fat: 5.6g| Carbs: 6.1g| Fiber: 0.9g| Protein: 1.7g

---

Strawberry Mousse

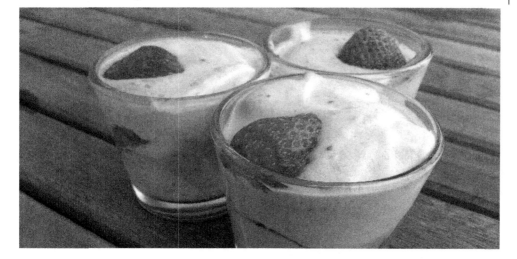

Ingredients

- 1½ C. fresh strawberries, hulled
- 1 2/3 C. chilled unsweetened coconut milk
- 2 tsp. powdered Erythritol
- 1 tsp. organic vanilla extract

Directions

1. In a food processor, add all the ingredients and pulse until smooth.

2. Transfer into serving bowls and serve.

Per Serving:

Calories: 114| Fat: 9.3g| Carbs: 4.5g| Fiber: 0.7g| Protein: 1.1g

Blueberry Scones

Servings: 08
Prep time: 15 mins
Cooking Time: 22 mins

Ingredients

- 1 tbsp. ground flaxseeds
- 3 tbsp. water
- 1 C. blanched almond flour
- ¼ C. coconut flour
- 3 tbsp. granulated Erythritol
- ½ tsp. baking powder
- 1/8 tsp. salt
- ¼ C. unsweetened almond milk
- 2 tbsp. coconut oil, melted
- 1 tsp. vanilla extract
- ½ C. fresh blueberries

Directions

1. Preheat your oven to 350 °F. Line a baking sheet with parchment paper.
2. For scones: in a large-sized bowl, add the ground flaxseeds and water and mix until seeds are absorbed completely.
3. Set aside for about 5 minutes.
4. Add the flours, Erythritol, baking powder and salt in a bowl and mix until well combined.
5. In the bowl of the flaxseed mixture, add the almond milk, coconut oil and vanilla extract and beat until well combined.
6. Add the flour mixture and mix until a pliable dough forms.
7. Gently fold in the blueberries.
8. Arrange the dough onto the prepared baking sheet and with your hands, pat into 1-inch thick circle.
9. Carefully cut the circle into 8 equal-sized wedges.
10. Now, arrange the scones in a single layer about 1-inch apart
11. Bake for approximately 18-22 minutes or until the top becomes golden brown
12. Remove from oven and place the baking sheet onto a wire rack to cool completely before serving.

Per Serving:

Calories: 128| Fat: 11.1g| Carbs: 3.9g| Fiber: 2.2g| Protein: 0.2g

Oat & Walnut Brownies

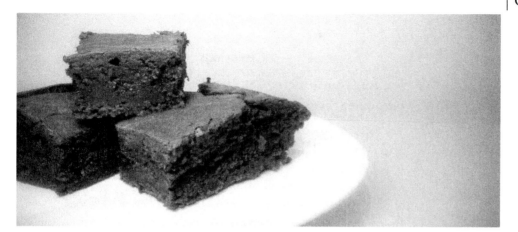

Ingredients

- Non-stick cooking spray
- 2 tbsp. flaxseed meal
- 6 tbsp. water
- 2 C. gluten-free oats
- 1 C. whole-wheat flour
- 2 scoops unsweetened protein powder
- ¾ C. Erythritol
- ¼ C. cacao powder
- 1 tsp. baking soda
- 1 tsp. salt
- 2/3 C. unsweetened applesauce
- 2/3 C. olive oil
- 1 tsp. organic vanilla extract
- 1/8 C. walnuts, chopped
- 1 tbsp. unsweetened dark chocolate chips

Directions

1. Preheat your oven to 350 °F. Grease a 9x13-inch baking dish with cooking spray.
2. In a small-sized bowl, add the flaxseed meal and water and mix well.
3. Set aside for about 5 minutes.
4. In a large-sized bowl, blend together the oats, flour, Erythritol, protein powder, cocoa powder, baking soda and salt.
5. Add the applesauce, oil, vanilla extract and flax mixture and mix until a thick dough forms.
6. Fold in the walnuts and chocolate chips.
7. Place the mixture into the prepared baking dish and with your hands, press to smooth the surface.
8. Bake for approximately 15-18 minutes.
9. Remove from oven and place onto a wire rack to cool completely.
10. Cut into equal-sized brownies and serve.

Per Serving:

Calories: 247| Fat: 14.9g| Carbs: 21.9g| Fiber: 3.3g| Protein: 8.7g

Carrot Pudding

Servings: 04
Prep time: 15 mins
Cooking Time: 31 mins

Ingredients

- 2-2½ C. unsweetened almond milk
- ¼ C. raw cashews
- 1 tbsp. olive oil
- 2 C. carrots, peeled and shredded
- 1-3 tbsp. Erythritol
- ¼ tsp. ground cardamom
- Pinch of ground cinnamon
- Pinch of salt
- 3 tbsp. mixed nuts, chopped

Directions

1. In a high-power blender, add almond milk and cashews and pulse until smooth and creamy.
2. Heat oil in a wok over medium heat and cook the carrots for about 5-6 minutes, stirring occasionally.
3. Add in the almond milk and cook for about 10 minutes, stirring occasionally.
4. Reduce heat to medium-low and stir in the Erythritol, cardamom, cinnamon and salt
5. Add in the nuts and raisins and cook partially covered for about 10-15 minutes, stirring occasionally.
6. Serve warm..

Per Serving:
Calories: 164| Fat: 13g| Carbs: 10.9g| Fiber: 2.6g| Protein: 3.3g

---

Coconut Macaroons

Servings: 12
Prep time: 15 mins
Cooking Time: 16 mins

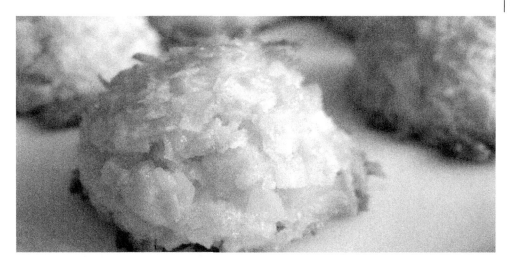

Ingredients

Directions

- 1¼ C. unsweetened coconut, shredded finely
- ¼ C. blanched almond flour
- ¼ C. maple syrup
- 3 tbsp. coconut oil

1. Preheat your oven to 350 °F. Line a baking sheet with parchment paper.
2. In a food processor, add all the ingredients and pulse until a thick, sticky mixture forms.
3. With a scooper, place the balls onto the prepared baking sheet about 1 inch apart.
4. Bake for 12-16 minutes until golden.
5. Remove from oven and immediately transfer the macaroons onto a wire rack to cool completely before serving.

Per Serving:
Calories: 90| Fat: 7.3g| Carbs: 6.2g| Fiber: 1g| Protein: 0.8g

Peanut Butter Fudge

Servings: 16
Prep time: 15 mins

Ingredients

- 1½ C. creamy, salted peanut butter
- 1/3 C. coconut oil
- 2/3 C. powdered Erythritol
- ¼ C. unsweetened protein powder
- 1 tsp. organic vanilla extract

Directions

1. In a small-sized saucepan, add peanut butter and coconut oil over low heat and cook until melted and smooth.
2. Add Erythritol and protein powder and mix until smooth.
3. Remove from heat and stir in vanilla extract.
4. Place the fudge mixture into a baking paper-lined 8x8-inch baking dish evenly and with a spatula, smooth the top surface.
5. Freeze for about 30-45 minutes or until set completely.
6. Carefully transfer the fudge onto a cutting board with the help of parchment paper.
7. Cut the fudge into equal-sized squares and serve.

Per Serving:
Calories: 207| Fat: 16.6g| Carbs: 9.5g| Fiber: 3g| Protein: 6.5g

Apple Crisp

Servings: 08

Prep time: 15 mins

Cooking Time: 20 mins

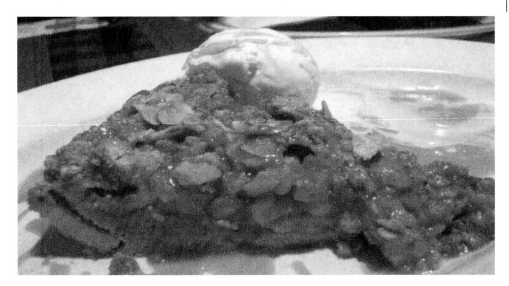

Ingredients

For Filling

- Non-stick cooking spray
- 2 large apples, peeled, cored, and chopped
- 2 tbsp. water
- 2 tbsp. fresh apple juice
- ¼ tsp. ground cinnamon

For Topping

- ½ C. gluten-free quick rolled oats
- ¼ C. unsweetened coconut flakes
- 2 tbsp. pecans, chopped
- ½ tsp. ground cinnamon
- ¼ C. water

Directions

1. Preheat your oven to 300 °F. Lightly grease a baking dish with cooking spray.
2. For filling: add all of the ingredients in a large-sized bowl and gently mix. Set aside.
3. For topping: add all of the ingredients in another bowl and mix well.
4. Place the filling mixture into the prepared baking dish then spread the topping over the filling mixture evenly.
5. Bake for approximately 20 minutes or until the top becomes golden brown.
6. Serve warm.

Per Serving:

Calories: 116| Fat: 4.1g| Carbs: 19.8g| Fiber: 2.9g| Protein: 1.5g

Brown Rice Pudding

Servings: 06

Prep time: 10 mins

Cooking Time: 25 mins

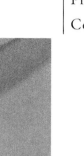

Ingredients

- 1½ C. cooked brown rice, lightly mashed
- 3 C. unsweetened almond milk
- 2 C. unsweetened coconut milk
- 1/3 C. Erythritol
- 2 tbsp. pistachios, crushed
- 2 tbsp. almonds, sliced
- ¼ tsp. ground cardamom
- Pinch of saffron strands

Directions

1. In a heavy-bottomed saucepan, add all ingredients except for saffron over medium-high heat and bring to a boil.
2. Adjust the heat to medium-low and cook for about 20 minutes, stirring occasionally.
3. Remove from heat and stir in saffron.
4. Serve warm or chilled.

Per Serving:

Calories: 272| Fat: 22.5g| Carbs: 16.9g| Fiber: 3g| Protein: 4g

---

Tapioca Pudding

Servings: 06

Prep time: 10 mins

Cooking Time: 35 mins

Ingredients

- 6 C. water, divided
- 1½ lb. taro, peeled and cut into ½ inch pieces

Directions

1. In a medium-sized pan, add 4 C. of water and taro over high heat and bring to a boil.
2. Adjust the heat to medium and cook for about 20

- ½ C. tapioca pearls
- 1 (13¾-oz.) can unsweetened coconut milk
- 1 C. Erythritol

minutes.

3. Remove from heat and drain the water.
4. With a fork, mash the taro pieces slightly
5. Meanwhile, in a small-sized pan, add remaining water and bring to a boil.
6. Stir in the tapioca and cook for about 6 minutes.
7. Remove from heat and set the pan aside, covered for about 10-15 minutes, or until the pearls are translucent.
8. Through a colander, strain the tapioca and rinse under cold running water.
9. Return the tapioca into the pan with coconut, taro and Erythritol and mix well.
10. Place the pan over medium heat and cook for about 2-3 minutes, stirring continuously.
11. Remove from heat and set aside to cool slightly.
12. Serve warm.

Per Serving:
Calories: 219| Fat: 1.2g| Carbs: 51g| Fiber: 6.2g| Protein: 0.6g

SMOOTHIES

Recipes

By: Lara Rush

Avocado Smoothie

Servings: 02
Prep time: 10 mins

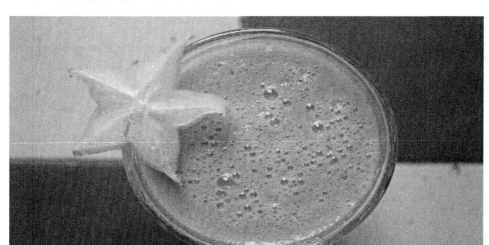

Ingredients

- 1 medium avocado, peeled, pitted and chopped
- 1 tsp. fresh lime zest, grated freshly
- 1 tbsp. fresh lime juice
- 2 tsp. maple syrup
- 1½ C. filtered water
- ¼ C. ice cubes

Directions

1. Add all the ingredients in a high-power blender and pulse until creamy.
2. Pour the smoothie into two glasses and serve immediately.

Per Serving:

Calories: 163| Fat: 13.8g| Carbs: 10.8g| Fiber: 4.9g| Protein: 1.4g

---

Avocado & Lettuce Smoothie

Servings: 02
Prep time: 10 mins

Ingredients

- 1 avocado, peeled, pitted and chopped
- 2 C. fresh lettuce
- 1 small banana, peeled and sliced
- 1½ C. unsweetened almond milk

Directions

1. Add all the ingredients in a high-power blender and pulse until creamy.
2. Pour the smoothie into two glasses and serve immediately.

- ¼ C. ice cubes

Per Serving:

Calories: 167| Fat: 15.1g| Carbs: 8.1g| Fiber: 6.3g| Protein: 2.3g

Avocado & Kiwi Smoothie

Servings: 02

Prep time: 10 mins

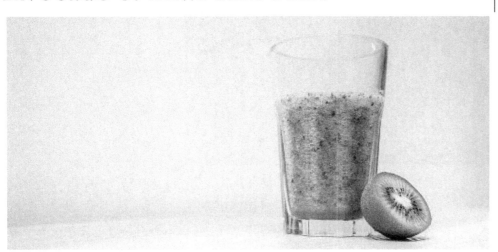

Ingredients

- 1 kiwi, peeled and chopped
- 1 small avocado, peeled, pitted and chopped
- 1 C. cucumber, peeled and chopped
- 2 C. fresh baby kale
- ¼ C. fresh mint leaves
- 2 C. filtered water
- ¼ C. ice cubes

Directions

1. Add all the ingredients in a high-power blender and pulse until creamy.
2. Pour the smoothie into two glasses and serve immediately.

Per Serving:

Calories: 185| Fat: 11.4g| Carbs: 20.3g| Fiber: 7g| Protein: 4.2g

Cucumber & Parsley Smoothie

Servings: 02

Prep time: 10 mins

Ingredients

- 2 C. cucumber, peeled and chopped

Directions

1. Add all the ingredients in a high-power blender and pulse until creamy.

- 2 C. fresh parsley
- 1 (1-inch) piece fresh ginger root, peeled and chopped
- 2 tbsp. fresh lime juice
- 4-6 drops liquid stevia
- 2 C. chilled filtered water

2. Pour the smoothie into two glasses and serve immediately.

Per Serving:

Calories: 40| Fat: 0.6g| Carbs: 8.1g| Fiber: 2.5g| Protein: 2.5g

---

Spinach & Blueberry Smoothie

Servings: 02
Prep time: 10 mins

Ingredients

- 1 C. fresh spinach
- ¾ C. fresh blueberries
- 1 tbsp. ground chia seeds
- 1 tbsp. ground flaxseeds
- ½ C. fat-free plain Greek yogurt
- 1 C. unsweetened almond milk
- ¼ C. ice cubes

Directions

1. Add all the ingredients in a high-power blender and pulse until creamy.
2. Pour the smoothie into two glasses and serve immediately.

Per Serving:

Calories: 115| Fat: 4.4g| Carbs: 16.1g| Fiber: 4.3g| Protein: 5.2g

---

Kale & Spinach Smoothie

Servings: 02
Prep time: 10 mins

Ingredients

- 2 C. fresh spinach
- 1 C. fresh kale, chopped
- 1 tbsp. peanut butter
- 1 tbsp. chia seeds
- 3-4 drops liquid stevia
- 1½ C. unsweetened almond milk

Directions

1. Add all the ingredients in a high-power blender and pulse until creamy.
2. Pour the smoothie into two glasses and serve immediately.

- ¼ C. ice cubes

Per Serving:

Calories: 115| Fat: 8g| Carbs: 9.2g| Fiber: 3.6g| Protein: 5.4g

---

Kale & Raspberry Smoothie

Servings: 02
Prep time: 10 mins

Ingredients

- 2 C. fresh kale, trimmed and chopped
- 1 C. fresh raspberries
- 1 tbsp. chia seeds
- 4-6 drops liquid stevia
- 1½ C. unsweetened almond milk
- ¼ C. ice cubes

Directions

1. Add all the ingredients in a high-power blender and pulse until creamy.
2. Pour the smoothie into two glasses and serve immediately.

Per Serving:

Calories: 110| Fat: 4.3g| Carbs: 17.3g| Fiber: 7g| Protein: 4.2g

---

Spinach & Apple Smoothie

Servings: 02
Prep time: 10 mins

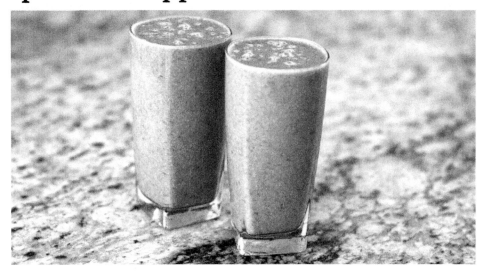

Ingredients

- 1 green apple, peeled, cored and chopped
- 2 C. fresh baby spinach leaves
- ½ C. fresh mint leaves
- 1 tbsp. fresh lime juice
- 1½ C. coconut water
- ½ C. ice cubes

Directions

1. Add all the ingredients in a high-power blender and pulse until creamy.
2. Pour the smoothie into two glasses and serve immediately.

Per Serving:

Calories: 110| Fat: 0.9g| Carbs: 25.1g| Fiber: 6.9g| Protein: 3.2g

Greens & Strawberry Smoothie

Servings: 02
Prep time: 10 mins

Ingredients

- 1 C. fresh strawberries, hulled and sliced
- 1 C. fresh kale, trimmed and chopped
- 1 C. fresh spinach, chopped
- ½ cucumber, peeled and chopped
- 1½ C. unsweetened almond milk
- ¼ C. ice cubes

Directions

1. Add all the ingredients in a high-power blender and pulse until creamy.
2. Pour the smoothie into two glasses and serve immediately.

Per Serving:

Calories: 84| Fat: 3g| Carbs: 13.8g| Fiber: 3.4g| Protein: 3.2g

Broccoli & Celery Smoothie

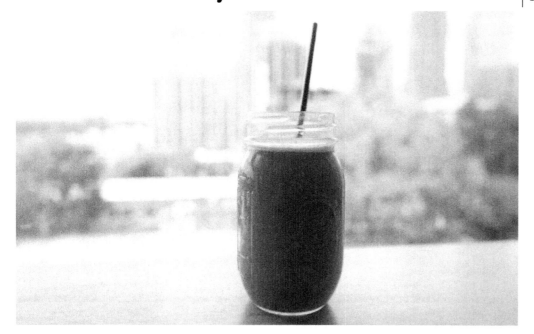

Ingredients

- 1 C. broccoli florets, chopped
- 1½ C. celery, chopped
- 1 banana, peeled and sliced
- ½ C. fresh parsley, chopped
- ¼ C. fresh basil leaves
- 1 C. filtered water
- ½ C. ice cubes

Directions

1. Add all the ingredients in a high-power blender and pulse until creamy.
2. Pour the smoothie into two glasses and serve immediately.

Per Serving:

Calories: 94| Fat: 0.7g| Carbs: 21.3g| Fiber: 5.1g| Protein: 3.6g

6 WEEK MEAL PLAN

Week 1:

Day 1:
Breakfast: Avocado Smoothie
Lunch: Shrimp Lettuce Wraps
Snack: Spiced Almonds
Dinner: Barley & Beans Soup

Day 2:
Breakfast: Eggs with Tomatoes
Lunch: Green Beans Salad
Snack: Hummus Bites
Dinner: Braised Chicken Thighs

Day 3:
Breakfast: Apple Porridge
Lunch: Beans & Walnut Burgers
Snack: Carrot Cookies
Dinner: Stuffed Steak

Day 4:
Breakfast: Oat Waffles
Lunch: Pumpkin Soup
Snack: Salted Edamame
Dinner: Tuna with Olives

Day 5:
Breakfast: Poached Eggs with Toast
Lunch: Tofu with Kale
Snack: Chickpeas Fries
Dinner: Maple Glazed Salmon

Day 6:
Breakfast: Spinach Muffins
Lunch: Turkey Meatloaf
Snack: Carrot Hummus
Dinner: Chickpeas & Quinoa Salad

Day 7:
Breakfast: Oats & Quinoa Granola
Lunch: Lentil & Rice Loaf
Snack: Fruity Oat Bites
Dinner: Chicken & Kale Stew

Week 2:

Day 1:
Breakfast: Baked Oatmeal
Lunch: Berries & Arugula Salad
Snack: Glazed Cashews
Dinner: Chicken with Capers Sauce

Day 2:
Breakfast: French Toast
Lunch: Scallops with Spinach
Snack: Brownie Bites
Dinner: Lentils with Kale

Day 3:
Breakfast: Carrot Muffins
Lunch: Stuffed Zucchini
Snack: Nuts & Seeds Bars
Dinner: Beef & Veggie Soup

Day 4:
Breakfast: Beet & Strawberry Smoothie Bowl
Lunch: Shrimp Lettuce Wraps
Snack: Tofu & Veggie Gazpacho
Dinner: Pasta & Beans Soup

Day 5:
Breakfast: Blueberry Pancakes
Lunch: Tofu with Kale
Snack: Spiced Cookies
Dinner: Chicken Salad

Day 6:
Breakfast: Mushrooms & Egg Scramble
Lunch: Chicken Burgers
Snack: Chickpeas Fries
Dinner: Stuffed Salmon

Day 7:
Breakfast: Blueberry Chia Pudding
Lunch: Garlicky Shrimp
Snack: Brussels Sprout Chips
Dinner: Veggie Stew

Week 3:

Day 1:
Breakfast: Veggie Frittata
Lunch: Chicken Lettuce Wraps
Snack: Chocolate Oat Bites
Dinner: Chickpeas & Spinach Stew

Day 2:
Breakfast: Nuts & Seeds Cereal
Lunch: Cucumber & Tomato Salad
Snack: Spiced Almonds
Dinner: Tuna with Olives

Day 3:
Breakfast: Greens & Strawberry Smoothie
Lunch: Shrimp with Kale
Snack: Chickpeas Fries
Dinner: Braised Beef

Day 4:
Breakfast: Overnight Oatmeal
Lunch: Mushrooms with Bok Choy
Snack: Cranberry Bars
Dinner: Chicken with Capers Sauce

Day 5:
Breakfast: Avocado Toast
Lunch: Scallops with Broccoli
Snack: Fruity Oat Bites
Dinner: Lentil Salad

Day 6:
Breakfast: Kale & Cheddar Omelet
Lunch: Broccoli Soup
Snack: Glazed Cashews
Dinner: Braised Chicken Thighs

Day 7:
Breakfast: Berries Yogurt Bowl

Lunch: Beans & Walnut Burgers
Snack: Carrot Cookies
Dinner: Stuffed Steak

Week 4:

Day 1:
Breakfast: Poached Eggs with Toast
Lunch: Green Beans Salad
Snack: Salted Edamame
Dinner: Braised Beef

Day 2:
Breakfast: Oat Waffles
Lunch: Shrimp Lettuce Wraps
Snack: Nuts & Seeds Bars
Dinner: Barley & Beans Soup

Day 3:
Breakfast: Mushrooms & Egg Scramble
Lunch: Turkey Meatloaf
Snack: Tofu & Veggie Gazpacho
Dinner: Stuffed Salmon

Day 4:
Breakfast: Oats & Quinoa Granola
Lunch: Beef Burgers
Snack: Carrot Cookies
Dinner: Barley & Veggies Pilaf

Day 5:
Breakfast: Apple Porridge
Lunch: Tofu with Kale
Snack: Carrot Hummus
Dinner: Chicken with Veggies

Day 6:
Breakfast: French Toast
Lunch: Stuffed Zucchini
Snack: Hummus Bites
Dinner: Parmesan Tilapia

Day 7:
Breakfast: Simple Bread
Lunch: Scallops with Broccoli
Snack: Brownie Bites

Dinner: Lentil Salad

Week 5:

Day 1:
Breakfast: Spinach & Apple Smoothie
Lunch: Mushrooms with Bok Choy
Snack: Tofu & Veggie Gazpacho
Dinner: Braised Chicken Thighs

Day 2:
Breakfast: Baked Oatmeal
Lunch: Apple & Pear Salad
Snack: Brussels Sprout Chips
Dinner: Maple Glazed Salmon

Day 3:
Breakfast: Eggs with Tomatoes
Lunch: Lentil & Rice Loaf
Snack: Spiced Cookies
Dinner: Chicken Salad

Day 4:
Breakfast: Spinach Muffins
Lunch: Shrimp with Kale
Snack: Glazed Cashews
Dinner: Veggie Stew

Day 5:
Breakfast: Carrot Muffins
Lunch: Berries & Arugula Salad
Snack: Chocolate Oat Bites
Dinner: Braised Beef

Day 6:
Breakfast: Nuts & Seeds Cereal
Lunch: Pumpkin Soup
Snack: Cranberry Bars
Dinner: Chicken & Kale Stew

Day 7:
Breakfast: Blueberry Chia Pudding
Lunch: Chicken Burgers
Snack: Salted Edamame
Dinner: Lentils with Kale

Week 6:

Day 1:
Breakfast: Kale & Cheddar Omelet
Lunch: Beef Burgers
Snack: Nuts & Seeds Bars
Dinner: Chickpeas & Quinoa Salad

Day 2:
Breakfast: Simple Bread
Lunch: Broccoli Soup
Snack: Brownie Bites
Dinner: Chicken with Veggies

Day 3:
Breakfast: Overnight Oatmeal
Lunch: Garlicky Shrimp
Snack: Salted Edamame
Dinner: Pasta & Beans Soup

Day 4:
Breakfast: Avocado Toast
Lunch: Mushrooms with Bok Choy
Snack: Brussels Sprout Chips
Dinner: Parmesan Tilapia

Day 5:
Breakfast: Cucumber & Lettuce Smoothie
Lunch: Scallops with Spinach
Snack: Carrot Hummus
Dinner: Barley & Veggie Pilaf

Day 6:
Breakfast: Veggie Frittata
Lunch: Cucumber & Tomato Salad
Snack: Chickpeas Fries
Dinner: Beef & Veggie Soup

Day 7:
Breakfast: Berries Yogurt Bowl
Lunch: Chicken Lettuce Wraps
Snack: Spiced Almonds
Dinner: Chickpeas & Spinach Stew

CONCLUSION

A diabetic diet is a way of eating that helps to keep blood sugar levels under control. There are many different types of diabetes, but all have one common goal: to maintain blood sugar within the target range. Achieving and maintaining this goal can be accomplished in several ways, including by following a diabetic diet.

There are also plenty of great recipes for meals and snacks that fit into a diabetic diet plan. And if you need some ideas or inspiration, check out our list of top 10 diabetes superfoods!

The best way to determine which foods work best for you is to experiment and find what works for your individual needs and preferences. But no matter what you choose to eat, always remember to consult with your doctor or health care professional before making any big changes to your diet.

INDEX

Printed in Great Britain
by Amazon

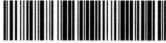